ANY GIVEN

MONDAY

Sports Injuries and How to Prevent Them,
for Athletes, Parents, and Coaches—
Based on My Life in Sports Medicine

Dr. James R. Andrews
with Don Yaeger

Scribner
New York   London   Toronto   Sydney   New Delhi

SCRIBNER
A Division of Simon & Schuster, Inc.
1230 Avenue of the Americas
New York, NY 10020

First Scribner trade paperback edition January 2014

SCRIBNER and design are registered trademarks of The Gale Group, Inc., used under license by Simon & Schuster, Inc., the publisher of this work.

For information about special discounts for bulk purchases, please contact Simon & Schuster Special Sales at 1-866-506-1949 or business@simonandschuster.com.

The Simon & Schuster Speakers Bureau can bring authors to your live event. For more information or to book an event, contact the Simon & Schuster Speakers Bureau at 1-866-248-3049 or visit our website at www.simonspeakers.com.

Designed by Carla Jayne Jones

Manufactured in the United States of America

10 9 8 7 6 5 4 3 2 1

Library of Congress Control Number: 2012028374

ISBN 978-1-4516-6708-0
ISBN 978-1-4516-6709-7 (pbk)
ISBN 978-1-4516-6710-3 (ebook)

"The UCL Procedure Revisited: The Procedure I Use" by James R. Andrews, Patrick W. Jost, and E. Lyle Cain (American Sports Medicine Institute, Birmingham, AL) is a forthcoming publication by AOSSM. Reprinted by Permission of SAGE Publications, Inc.

A. D. Faigenbaum and L. Meaders. "A Coaches Dozen: 12 Fundamental Principles for Building Young, Healthy Athletes." *Strength and Conditioning Journal* 2010;32(2):99–101. Used by permission.

I dedicate this book to my wonderful wife, Jenelle; to all our children, Andy, Amy, Archie, Ashley, Amber, and Abby; and also to my grandkids, who have stood by me and supported me throughout my entire career. They have been instrumental in helping me sort out my priorities in life. Number one is my faith and a close second is my family. Next, my career and profession, which has been a wonderful lifetime journey.

I also dedicate the chapters on guidelines for prevention of injuries in youth sports to all the athletes whom I have been so privileged to treat and hopefully help. Being able to witness these individuals accomplish their goals not only in sports but in life in general is truly the joy and inspiration for my continued journey.

I would like to express my gratitude to my business administrator, H. Michael Immel; Lanier Johnson, the executive director of our American Sports Medicine Institute (ASMI); and all of the many other staff members, secretaries, nurses, therapists, athletic trainers, and researchers who as a team have made my life so successful and enjoyable.

From a legacy standpoint thanks so very much to all of the sports medicine fellows whom I have trained for challenging me and stimulating me to be the very best I could be. Thanks especially to Lyle Cain, MD; Jeff Dugas, MD; and Roger Ostrander, MD—my former fellows and now associates—for all they do in establishing my continued legacy.

I also dedicate this work to Don Yaeger and his staff, who were an incredible joy to work with.

—Dr. James Andrews

To my sister Nani. I admire you for all you've fought through to achieve great things. Keep the faith!

—Don Yaeger

Contents

Contents

ANY GIVEN MONDAY

Introduction
What Is the Point of This Book?

Why, after nearly forty years of practicing medicine and preparing for inevitable retirement, would I want to write a book? And since the focus of my practice for the majority of my career has been on adults, why would I choose to write a book about *youth* sports injuries?

The reasons are simple but tragic. I am writing this book because it absolutely needs to be written to help curb the growing epidemic that is endangering our most athletically talented children, adolescents, and young adults. I want to make sure that parents, grandparents, coaches, trainers, and all medical personnel are taking the steps now to maximize the opportunities for the next generation of young athletes. This book is intended to do just that: to raise awareness of the most common youth sports injuries and the best ways to prevent them, while explaining the most constructive ways to build a child's potential. My hope is to educate all adults on how to protect an active child already involved in organized sports and how to select the best activities and safest exercises for a child who is looking to get physically fit.

Juvenile obesity (and the health risks brought on by the condition, such as diabetes and cardiovascular disease) has captured a great deal of media and political attention in recent years, and poor dietary choices and a more sedentary lifestyle are often to blame.

But what about the children at the other end of the spectrum: the ones who are not only physically active but also follow a strict athletic training regimen and dedicate dozens of hours every week to exercise and activity? The serious health risks facing those children are often overlooked or simply shrugged off as "just part of growing up." But the truth is that youth sports injuries are an epidemic in American society, and we can do more to combat them.

Every year, more than three and a half million children under the age of fourteen require medical treatment for injuries incurred while participating in team or individual sports, and this number is on the rise. Over the past fifteen years, children have gone from being a rarity on my operating table to constituting nearly half of all my patients. More than one-fifth of all traumatic brain injuries in children are the direct result of athletic activity. Almost one-half of all sports injuries in adolescents stem from overuse, in which specific muscles and joints are damaged due to repetitive motion as part of athletic training or conditioning.

Yet despite these startling statistics, sports injuries are largely preventable, especially in children and adolescents. Even something as seemingly harmless as overuse of a joint or muscle can have a dramatic impact on future athletic ability, and even basic functions of movement and control. Both the short-term and long-term repercussions need to be considered when a child begins participating in any kind of sport.

Over the course of my nearly forty-year career, I have been the go-to surgeon for high-profile professional athletes such as Roger Clemens, Albert Pujols, Charles Barkley, Scottie Pippen, Kerri Strug, Jack Nicklaus, Raymond Floyd, Jerry Pate, Troy Aikman, Drew Brees, Brett Favre, Bo Jackson, Emmitt Smith, Terrell Owens, Sam Bradford, Matthew Stafford, and both Manning brothers, just to name a few. My goal has always been not only to return these great sports icons to the top of their game but also to help spread awareness of the causes and prevention of potentially career-ending injuries. *Any Given Monday* refers to the major consultation day in my clinic, when many of America's premier athletes, fresh off broadcast TV, arrive at the Andrews Clinic in Birmingham, Alabama, or at the Andrews Institute for Orthopaedics & Sports Medicine in Gulf Breeze, Florida, for an examination of any injuries from their weekend matchups.

At least once a week, concerned parents will come into my clinic to inquire about their child's hurt shoulder, swollen elbow, or aching knee and how that injury could affect his or her athletic participation. As part of the exam, I will ask the parents to detail the child's practice schedule for the past month and year on a blackboard in the examination room so that we can look at it together. More often than not, the intensity, amount, and duration of the exercises are staggering—sometimes they are actually comparable to the training regimen of a pro. I sit down with the family and try to make them understand the potentially irreversible damage that such a schedule can do to a growing body; then we discuss better options. I want parents to seriously consider the implications of putting a twelve-year-old through the same paces as a twenty-five-year-old. Many times they have no idea as to the extent of the injury that their child is suffering; the focus of many parents and coaches is simply on pushing the child to achieve at the highest level possible for college opportunities or to gain a big break into the professional realm. What they often don't seem to realize is that if a child's body is overworked at an early age, he or she might not be able to stay in that sport long enough to make it to high school varsity, let alone to the elite level they so desperately desire. Families come to me to put their dream back together, but I want to make sure that parents and coaches understand how to prevent those dreams from shattering in the first place. Those adults have the child's best interest at heart, but most do not fully understand the risk factors at play in a specific sport.

This dangerous trend is continuing to rise year after year, while the average age of the patients on my table continues to drop. Baseball, in particular, posts some of the highest numbers in terms of serious injuries in youth sports. Recently, in a single day, I completed eight Tommy John surgeries—an operation to repair an injured elbow. Two of my patients were major league pitchers, two pitched for college teams, and *four* were high schoolers ranging in age from fourteen to seventeen. The following day, I took a photograph of them all together, their arms in splints and ice bags on their shoulders. It was a remarkable day because it reminded me how widespread the problem of professional-level injuries has become, even at the teenage level.

This book will pull from the hundreds of anecdotes and examples I have collected over the past four decades to highlight the types of injuries that are common in athletics; the consequences of childhood injuries; and the advice, treatment, and rehabilitation plans I have prescribed for many of the sports stars you see dominating the field or court every week. Because of the real-life experiences of sports figures who have been on my operating table and now are outspoken advocates for youth sports injury prevention, this book offers readers a personal connection to the headliners who promote this important cause.

Additionally, *Any Given Monday* provides a reference guide to the twenty-eight most popular youth sports, outlining the health concerns most common to each, how best to treat them, and how to prevent them from happening again—or from happening in the first place. It also addresses the various myths and misconceptions surrounding juvenile orthopedic sports medicine and serves as an overall guide to raising healthy, injury-free children and young adults.

I want to take a moment to speak specifically to the grandparents who might be reading this book. I want to thank you for the interest you've taken in the lives of the grandchildren you love, and I hope you know that the role of grandparents in looking out for young athletes is now more important than ever. In some cases, grandparents are also primary caregivers, which is a serious undertaking. Athletics may have changed since you were in high school—both the types of sports that are now popular as well as the style or roughness of play. Safety equipment and rules may also have undergone some changes. I hope that this book will help you to gain a better understanding of current trends, rules, and modes of thinking surrounding youth sports.

For those grandparents, I also believe that the information presented here will help you feel more connected to the world of training and competition in which your grandchild is involved. But even more than that, I hope it helps empower you to voice any concerns you may have. Very often in my practice, I have seen that it was the grandparents who first recognized an overuse injury or burnout in a child or teen. Sometimes the parents are too close to the situation and so wrapped up in carpools, prepping postpractice snacks, and making sure that homework is completed after practice that they miss some of the warning signs right in front of them. Other times, a child might admit to a grandparent that he is experiencing pain or exhaustion due to participation in a certain sport but doesn't want to tell his parents for fear of disappointing them. If grandparents sense that a grandchild is being overworked or overcommitted, I urge you to express your worries and your desire to see your grandchild live as healthily as possible. By gently explaining the long-term risks of year-round leagues and overuse injuries, you might be able to help protect the growing joints, muscles, and bones of the young athlete's body, enabling him to maximize his talent as he grows older.

Because of the work conducted at my clinics in Birmingham and Gulf Breeze by my highly talented staff of physicians, surgeons, physical therapists, athletic trainers, and other experts, in 2010 *Sports Illustrated* named me one of the forty most influential people in the National Football League. It was an honor I both greatly appreciated and deeply regretted. It is my sincere desire to see a generation of athletes grow up knowing how to care properly for their bodies, how to explore and grow their talent in the most effective way, and how to reduce the need for work such as mine through proactive treatment.

As part of my effort to see this goal through to reality, all of my personal proceeds from *Any Given Monday* will go directly to the STOP (Sports Trauma and Overuse Prevention) Sports Injuries Campaign I helped to initiate as president of the American Orthopaedic Society for Sports Medicine (AOSSM) during 2009 and 2010. Together with members of our "Council of Champions"—including Hank Aaron, Bonnie Blair, Shaquille O'Neal, Bart Starr, Matthew Stafford, and industrialist Jim Justice, among many others—I have appeared on numerous public service announcements and talk shows on networks ranging from ESPN to HBO. To learn more, please visit the STOP website at www.stopsportsinjuries.org.

But lest this come across as a thinly veiled self-promotion, I need to stress that this book is not about me. My life and my career have never been an "I" statement but a "we" situation!

Introduction

There are doctors out there doing far more to saves lives and combat serious illnesses than I have ever done or will ever do. There are many surgeons in my own field of orthopedics who are working continually to improve the lives of men, women, and children with devastating injuries. There are specialists dedicated to helping wounded veterans learn to adapt to life with prosthetic limbs and others who are focused on helping children with physical birth defects achieve full, enriching lives. These are the real heroes of the medical field: the doctors, nurses, and therapists who are helping one person at a time reclaim his or her birthright of "life, liberty, and the pursuit of happiness."

But me? I have just been fortunate enough to work with famous people who throw or bat around a ball for a living.

Of course, athletes have every right to those goals as do the rest of us, but sometimes it seems a little backward that people know my name because they've seen it mentioned in articles or interviews with A-list sports celebrities and not because I've cured anything or changed the world for the better.

I think that's important to state at the opening of this book. While I am writing about some of my experiences and philosophies, this book is not intended to celebrate my accomplishments or contributions to the world of sports medicine. Anything I share about my life and career is intended to introduce myself to the reader and establish a sense of credibility for my recommendations.

It is my hope that the long-standing relationships I have had the privilege of sharing with many high-profile athletes will help to make this book an automatic and authoritative platform from which to reach parents, grandparents, coaches, and children with the message: "Safe on the playing field, out of the operating room."

It's time to put a stop to this pervasive problem that is, quite literally, crippling our children before they even have a chance to live their dreams—and to focus on the behaviors and practices that can help a child maximize his or her athletic potential.

If that is the goal you have for your child, then we have a great deal in common and a lot to discuss. I urge you to read on.

Part 1

Why It Matters

Chapter 1
The Epidemic

Approximately forty-five million children and adolescents are involved in organized athletics in the United States and, as I stated earlier, nearly three and a half million of them under the age of fourteen are treated for sports-related injuries each year, making athletics one of the leading health risks for children. The majority of injuries, of course, are relatively mild sprains, strains, and bruises, but a significant percentage will be more severe, with some even requiring hospitalization. What is even more troubling is that roughly 50 percent of all sports injuries are related to overuse, and studies show that at least 60 percent of overuse injuries can be prevented simply by employing a little common sense—and even more by taking just a few safety precautions. It must be the primary responsibility of the parents, grandparents, coaches, paramedical personnel, and young athletes themselves to help prevent these injuries the best they can.

These statistics are followed carefully by the American Sports Medicine Institute (ASMI) and the Andrews Research & Education Institute (AREI) in Gulf Breeze, two organizations of which I am the chairman. Each year, as new numbers come in, it is a sobering experience for many reasons. Injuries certainly reduce participation in sports and fitness activities, thus contributing to the childhood obesity epidemic as well as other social misgivings. Some injuries can be career ending or even life limiting well before the child or teen has had a chance to pursue his or her dreams. Even less serious injuries can have long-term implications, as damage to joints in childhood contributes exponentially to the chances of developing arthritis later in life. Additionally, there is no question that the evaluation, treatment, and rehabilitation of youth sports injuries is expensive and can lead to lost time and productivity at work for parents. Recent reports have placed the costs associated with youth sports injuries between $2.5 billion and $3 billion annually.

As stated above, many of these sports-related youth injuries are preventable through educational programs at the grassroots level. I will discuss some of the more common youth sports and associated injuries and provide some information related to their prevention, including rule changes, safety equipment, and preseason and in-season conditioning programs.

Our statistics at the American Sports Medicine Institute indicate a five- to seven-fold increase in injuries in youth sports since 2000. Further statistics show that in high school alone, each year some two million injuries result in five hundred thousand doctor visits and approximately thirty thousand hospitalizations for treatment. The statistics for certain sports are particularly troubling.

Cheerleading, for example, is out of control. There are three million young cheerleaders in the United States, ranging from squads of preteens at local cheer gyms, to approximately four hundred thousand at the high school level, to the college cheerleaders you see on TV, smiling and leaping on the sidelines at football and basketball games. The National Collegiate Athletic Association's (NCAA) medical reports indicate that of all the insurance monies spent on treatment for college athletes across roughly ninety sports, fully 25 percent is for cheerleading injuries. This might not seem as dramatic a number when compared to the 57 percent of NCAA medical expenses spent on football; however, football has ten times the participation of cheerleading. The rate of emergency room visits for cheerleaders at any level has increased sixfold since 1981. In 2008 alone, roughly thirty thousand young women and men landed in the ER as a result of injuries sustained while cheering. During the twenty-six years between 1982 and 2008, there were seventy-three catastrophic injuries reported in cheerleading, with two deaths. Gymnastics, which incorporates many of the same tumbling passes and boasts similar numbers of participants, had a total of nine catastrophic injuries during that same period. That's a pretty drastic difference. Clearly, something needs to be done to protect cheerleaders from increasingly common and increasingly serious injuries. Football, too, deserves a critical examination. In 2007 there were 920,000 players under the age of eighteen treated in emergency rooms for injuries.

One factor that contributes significantly to the rate of injury is specialization. In other words, children are pigeonholed into one sport fairly early on, which means that they have little variation in terms of the muscles and joints employed and skills practiced, which can lead to fatigue and a much higher rate of injury. And one of the main causes of early specialization is parents who stress the pursuit of one specific sport for the sake of gaining college scholarships and professional recruiting buzz. It should be noted, though, that the odds of a football player actually making it to the NFL—not as a starter or even taking the field at any point in his life, but just making it on a professional roster—is greater than 6,000 to 1.

I don't mean to come down too hard on parents here; after all, we all want the best possible opportunities for our children. And most parents are very responsible in the emphasis they place on pursuing sports. But at some point, there needs to be a reality check. Ambitious parents and coaches need to understand that encouraging a child's talent is one thing but controlling it or obsessing over it is quite another. Before you pin your future retirement plans on how well your child performs athletically, consider this: The National Federation of State High School Associations estimates that less than 0.1 percent of kids who participate in sports at school will receive a scholarship to continue that sport in college.

The American Orthopaedic Society for Sports Medicine (AOSSM) initiated the STOP Sports Injury Campaign in 2010 to prevent overuse and trauma injuries among young athletes. The STOP acronym, which stands for Sports Trauma and Overuse Prevention, makes clear the organization's intentions. As president of the society from 2009 to 2010, I expressed my desire to launch a national program for preventing injuries in youth sports. The AOSSM unanimously agreed that the time was right to begin our education campaign.

Founding partner organizations in the STOP Sports Injury Campaign include the American Academy of Orthopaedic Surgeons (AAOS), the American Academy of Pediatrics (AAP), the American Medical Society for Sports Medicine (AMSSM), the National Athletic Trainers' Association (NATA), the National Strength and Conditioning Association (NSCA), the Pediatric Orthopaedic Society of North America (POSNA), the Sports Physical Therapy Section of the American Physical Therapy Association (APTA), Safe Kids USA, and the Professional Baseball Athletic Trainers Society (PBATS). Today there are more than 250 other local and national organizations that have taken the pledge to prevent youth sports injuries at the grassroots level.

When it comes to sports injury prevention, we must establish a priority in basic research principles. The STOP program's mission is fourfold: Number one is to establish the extent of the problem. Number two is to identify the risk factors and the mechanism of the injuries. Number three is to develop preventive interventions. And number four is to evaluate the effects and results of those interventions from a scientific standpoint. The STOP program has all of these objectives in its mission and focus. The AOSSM has identified several areas of research that need to be undertaken to take prevention to a scientific conclusion and to be able to show definitive results.

The first high-priority proposal addresses the *prevention of anterior cruciate ligament (ACL) knee injuries in young female athletes,* who have a three to six times ACL injury rate when compared to their male counterparts. This study will emphasize "cutting" sports, which require a sudden change of direction or darting to one side while running, such as basketball, lacrosse, soccer, and volleyball. Cheerleading and gymnastics will also be included.

The second priority is the *prevention of repeated concussions and related complications.* Approximately two million to three million young athletes suffer concussions each year in America. A number of long-term studies have shown that repeated concussions have an impact on mental health later in life, especially among former athletes.

The third priority is related to *overuse injuries of the shoulder and elbow and their prevention in youth baseball and youth softball* for both pitchers and fielders. The number of young men and women who require surgical repair to their pitching arms because of overuse damage is on the rise. This is a serious problem and one that is especially close to my heart, as it is now one of the most common procedures I have to perform on young people. When I started in this career, I never imagined that it would become routine for a fifteen-year-old to have to undergo such drastic treatment.

In a study published in the September 2009 issue of the *American Journal of Sports Medicine,* researchers examined severe injuries broken down by specific sports and injury type. Researchers captured injury data during the 2005–06 and 2006–07 school years from one hundred nationally represented US high schools. Information was collected for various sports, including football, soccer, volleyball, basketball, wrestling, baseball, and softball. "Severe injury" was defined as any mishap that resulted in an athlete losing more than twenty-one days of sports participation; according to the study, over the course of those two years, severe injuries accounted for 14.9 percent of all high school sports–related injuries. After football injuries, the highest level of injury was reported in wrestling, followed by girls' basketball and girls' soccer. While no one was surprised that football emerged as number one, there were some unexpected findings. Among the directly comparable sports of soccer, basketball, and baseball/softball, girls actually sustained a higher severe injury rate than boys. There were also patterns in injury sites, with the knee sustaining a severe injury nearly 30 percent of the time, followed by the ankle at 12.3 percent and the shoulder at 10.9 percent. Additionally, 5 percent of the severe injuries recorded resulted directly from illegal player activity such as tripping or spear tackling. While ankle sprains still tend to be the most common "nonsevere" injury among young players, these findings highlighted the importance of finding ways to protect the knees from more traumatic damage, and suggested that not enough is being done to educate and protect young women athletes.

According to this very important and revealing article, future studies should focus on risk factors to develop prevention and intervention. Decreasing sports-related injuries is critical to keep kids playing sports long-term and minimizing the health care cost both to the family and to the health care system itself.

According to the National Federation of State High School Associations, some 7.34 million athletes now participate in high school sports programs, up from 5.2 million just ten years ago. The boy-to-girl ratio is not quite even, although the number of girls participating in sports is on the rise: The total numbers are approximately 4.32 million boys compared to 3.02 million girls, yet the number of serious injuries in many girls' sports is higher than the rate in comparable boys' sports. This is certainly a cause for concern.

In light of these statistics, I'd like to make some general recommendations for athletes of both genders that I will elaborate on in part 2's sports-specific chapters. The vast majority of sports medicine professionals, coaches, and trainers agree that training in the months prior to the sports season is critical to an athlete's success. The old saying "Preparation is ninety-nine percent of execution" is certainly true in the athletic arena. A very successful preseason strength and conditioning program will dramatically decrease the risk of both minor and major injuries. It is the responsibility of coaches in all youth sports to educate their players in proper *periodization* on a twelve-month basis in preparation for a season. That is, fitness must begin prior to the first day of practice, and, ideally, some form of physical fitness should be maintained year-round, with training increasing gradually two to three months before the season starts. Statistics show that the majority of injuries occur in the first few weeks of a sports season due to inadequate preseason preparation.

It is also critical for coaches and players to realize that there must be a balance between work and rest. A young athlete should not work out at peak levels twelve months out of the year—especially not with an eye toward specializing in a specific sport. Overtraining always increases the risk for injury, especially in growing bodies. Therefore, athletes should not neglect off-season training, specifically cross-training and participating in other sports. But they should also be willing to take off a few weeks or a month from intense exercise each year in order to allow their body to rest. Low-impact activity should be pursued during that time, but the body needs a chance to recover and repair itself from the constant wear and tear of training.

Coaches should also be aware that the US Consumer Product Safety Commission (CPSC) indicates that 62 percent of sports injuries occur during practice rather than in a game or match. This does make sense: although an athlete's adrenaline tends to be higher in competitive settings—contributing to more aggressive play—the vast majority of his or her time is spent in practice versus actual time going head-to-head with another team. For that reason, practices should always be well supervised for safety of technique as well as the intensity of the workout.

No matter the sport, it is important to focus on general conditioning and core stability, as well as overall cardiovascular fitness and endurance through long-duration, low-intensity workouts. Cross-training during the off-season is especially important when participating in a predominantly one-sided sport, such as baseball. By pursuing different types of sports, young athletes can develop more complete musculature and hone other athletic skills to avoid fatiguing a specific part of the body.

Young athletes, particularly those who have not yet gone through puberty, should avoid overtraining and overuse, as the body is not fully equipped to rebuild muscles following workouts. I recommend that younger athletes follow a simple 10 percent rule: do not increase weight, training activities, mileage, or pace by more than 10 percent a week. This prevents stressing the body beyond capacity by allowing it to rest, rebuild, and recover. In fact, increasing training intensity too quickly can actually *decrease* high-level athletic activity.

It is essential for coaches to understand the basic principles related to preparing an athlete for a season. Thanks to Avery D. Faigenbaum, EdD, at the College of New Jersey, and Larry Meadors, PhD, at Sports Spectrum Training, here's a list of twelve fundamentals for building young and healthy players, which the authors aptly entitle "The Coaches Dozen," originally published in *Strength and Conditioning Journal* in 2010:

1. Young athletes are not miniature adults.

2. Value preparatory conditioning.

3. Avoid sports specialization before adolescence.

4. Enhance physical literacy.

5. Better to undertrain than to overtrain.

6. Focus on positive education.

7. Maximize recovery.

8. It is not what you take, it is what you do.

9. Get connected.

10. Make a long-term commitment.

11. There are no secrets.

12. Never stop learning.

Coaches and parents alike should remember that sports are meant to be fun, while facilitating a young athlete's social development. Never push the training or make the competition so serious that the child feels stressed or comes to dread the activity. This can easily lead to burnout in the sport or in athletics in general. I also recommend avoiding "professionalism" in youth sports—that is, harping on how young athletes need to develop their talent if they ever want to make it in the pros, or obsessing over their training to the point of tunnel vision. Adolescents have plenty of time to develop into professional athletes if their talent and interest point them in that direction. Genetically, 99.9 percent of young athletes are not ready for such serious professionalism at a young age.

There are essentially two different types of injuries: acute injuries and overuse injuries. Acute injuries are the result of a single traumatic event. Common examples include wrist fractures, ankle sprains, shoulder dislocations, or hamstring muscle strains. Overuse injuries, on the other hand, usually occur over time, making them more challenging to diagnose and sometimes more difficult to treat, as the damage is often not as clearly defined as in acute injuries. They are usually a result of overtraining: repetitive microtrauma to tendons, bones, cartilage, and joints, such as shin splints or tennis elbow. Whenever an athlete trains for a sport, even as a child, he or she is trying to make the bones, muscles, tendons, and ligaments of the body stronger and more functional. Unfortunately, there is a very thin line between beneficial training and training that is ultimately detrimental to the body.

The process of breaking down and building up muscle has a fine balance as well. When is the soreness a good thing, meaning that the muscles were stretched and worked to the point of growing stronger? And when does it mean that the muscles were damaged and are struggling to repair themselves? Training errors tend to involve a rapid acceleration of the intensity, duration, or frequency of an activity. They are especially associated with specialization.

Parents, coaches, and athletes must remember that the goal is always to feel better, not worse. Although soreness is to be expected when working new muscles, and anyone is likely to feel winded when doing cardio conditioning, the pain should never be debilitating. A common philosophy in training for sports is that "more is better": in other words, if pitching a ball twenty times is good, pitching it forty times is twice as good. That's simply not true. "No pain, no gain" should have no place in youth sports. Young athletes should not participate with pain. Athletes should have an open dialogue with their coaches, parents, or other trusted adults regarding their pain patterns, as these may be early indications of overuse injuries.

When an imbalance between strength and flexibility occurs, the injury pattern for overuse injuries increases rapidly. Young athletes who are still developing and growing often have bony malalignment, which simply means that the bones are growing at a rate that temporarily puts them out of the normal position in relation to their joints. This condition makes young athletes even more prone to overuse injuries. Other factors include equipment (such as the type of running shoe or ballet shoe), whether the terrain is uneven, hard surfaces versus soft surfaces in training, and whether proper techniques are being taught and practiced. These are just a few of the reasons why expert, certified coaches are so important in bringing their knowledge and understanding of the safest and best possible practices to their teams.

Some guidelines for treating overuse injury include:

1. Cut back the intensity, duration, and frequency of an activity.

2. Adopt a hard/easy workout schedule to vary the intensity each day, and incorporate cross-training with other activities to maintain fitness levels.

3. Learn proper training and techniques from a qualified coach or athletic trainer.

4. Perform proper warm-up and cool-down activities before and after practicing. Flexibility stretches can be particularly helpful when combined with ballistic exercises that get the muscles ready for intense bursts of energy, such as squats or tossing a medicine ball. (See chapter 32 for more information and illustrations.)

5. Apply ice for minor aches and pains after any activity.

6. Use nonsteroidal anti-inflammatory medications (NSAIDs), such as aspirin, ibuprofen, and naproxen, as necessary. Communication between athletes, parents, and coaches is particularly important if symptoms persist, at which point a visit to a sports medicine specialist is in order.

7. Consult athletic trainers and physical therapists for guidelines about early recognition and treatment of suspected overuse.

Keeping our kids safe needs to be a team effort, with all involved parties pitching in. Parents, grandparents, coaches, trainers, and athletes should all work toward the brightest possible future for every young athlete: one that is healthy and active thanks to the safe decisions we make together now.

Chapter 2
What Is Sports Medicine?

We need to begin by talking about the importance of sports medicine and how it specifically targets the unique needs of athletes. A short definition of the practice is that it is "the care of the muscles, bones, and joints of athletically active individuals." But to understand the bigger picture, let's look at how it developed.

A Brief History of Sports Medicine

While sports medicine is one of the youngest fields of medical practice in many ways, it is also quite an ancient one. In the fifth century BC, a Greek-speaking physician from Thrace named Herodicus reportedly was the first team doctor and the father of sports medicine. He rendered his fundamental theories on the use of therapeutic exercises for maintaining health and treating disease, promoting not only a proper diet for peak athletic performance but also postworkout massages for the sake of rehabilitating sore muscles and joints. A gymnastics master as well as a practicing doctor, Herodicus mentored a number of younger athletes and physicians alike, such as Hippocrates, for whom is named the Hippocratic oath, which all physicians still take as part of their medical education and licensure.

An abundance of sports medicine theories have been put into practice in the intervening 2,500 years—some good, some bad, some with a lot of inconsistencies. The one fact that remains true throughout history is that athletic competition produces injuries, and some can be severe, career ending, and even deadly.

Sports medicine as we know it today really began in 1890 at Harvard Medical School. This was a logical place for the field to emerge, as Harvard University was the home of one of the nation's oldest and most competitive football teams. And even as the sport was taking off at the end of the nineteenth century, protective equipment still lagged behind: Helmets were not used widely until the 1920s, and even then were just thick leather caps rather than the carefully designed shells with face masks and strategic padding that are such an indispensable part of modern football. At Harvard, significant injuries following football games and other athletic competitions were recognized as unique health challenges; because of this, a program was instituted to educate the players about the need for personal fitness, proper gear, injury prevention, and the importance of rehabilitation. Team athletic trainers and therapists grew in importance along with the team physician. Modern sports medicine had begun.

For the next sixty years, Harvard continued to lead the way in developing this branch of medicine into a distinct field of practice. In 1899 Dr. E. A. Darling released a scientific report defining the physiological effects of strenuous athletic exercise and methods for decreasing related injuries. Five years later, team physician Dr. Edwin Nichols pushed for protective gear to be required in football.

The following year, in 1905, President Theodore Roosevelt formed the American Football Rules Committee. Led by Henry L. Williams, the AFRC laid the groundwork for what would eventually become the National Collegiate Athletic Association, the organization that now oversees sports programs at most US colleges and universities.

But sports medicine was growing not just in America. The term *sports physician* was first used in Germany in 1914. Nineteen thirty-three saw the formation of the Internationale de Medico-Sportive et Cientifique, which focused on medical practices for much of the athletic competition in Europe.

The first book on the subject was published in 1938 by Dr. Augustus Thorndike, a Harvard Medical School graduate, World War I veteran, and surgeon who began working with the Harvard University Athletic Department in 1926. His text, *Athletic Injuries: Prevention, Diagnosis and Treatment,* became the written authority for a generation of team doctors and trainers.

The 1940s and 1950s witnessed a huge increase in the number of scientific articles examining sports medicine in practice. In 1957 Harvard's team physician Dr. Thomas B. Quigley crafted what he called the "Athlete's Bill of Rights," a document that sparked a great deal of discussion as to the degree of medical care that athletes had a right to expect from their team.

By the start of the 1960s, University of Oklahoma team physician Dr. Don O'Donoghue's book *Treatment of Injuries to Athletes* had replaced Thorndike's book as the bible of sports medicine and helped to standardize training and approaches to injury treatment and prevention. Around that same time, in Columbus, Georgia, Dr. Jack C. Hughston, chairman of the American Medical Association's Sports Medicine Committee, worked to promote postgraduate courses in the field and encouraged more research on the subject, in effect, pushing it into mainstream medicine. Hughston also brought a team of physicians with him to high school football games on Friday nights, and then to college games at Auburn and other universities on Saturdays. Specialized athletic health care was becoming the rule rather than the exception.

The 1970s saw some of the most substantial changes in the field, however. The American Orthopaedic Society for Sports Medicine was born in 1972, with Don O'Donoghue as its first president. Along with the establishment of the AOSSM came its *Journal of Sports Medicine,* with Jack C. Hughston as the initial editor. It later became the *American Journal of Sports Medicine.*

Prior to 1978, there was little continuity or consistency in America with regard to how individual Olympic sports selected their own medical teams. The United States Olympic Committee launched a program to refine and regiment the care provided to Olympic athletes.

Even more significant during that same decade was the introduction of arthroscopy, a minimally invasive procedure in which a tiny camera inserted through a tiny incision in the body provided a view of internal injury. As technology improved, joint surgery was revolutionized. Suddenly knee injuries that had once been career ending could often be surgically repaired. Shoulder, elbow, ankle, hip, and wrist surgeries all offered new hope to injured athletes. This was the most important technical advancement in sports medicine in the last forty years, thanks to the late, great Dr. Robert Jackson, who brought the first arthroscope to North America from Japan.

The first sports medicine fellowships were established in the early 1970s. A fellow is a licensed doctor who is already qualified to be an orthopedic surgeon but is studying for another year to gain additional expertise in a subspecialty such as sports medicine. These fellowships were really apprenticeships that were individually organized, had various lengths of training, and were usually a one-on-one experience. At this time, thanks to the leadership from other collaborative sports medicine groups, the modern sports medicine team was born, which includes the following professionals: sports doctor, sports orthopedist-arthroscopist, athletic trainer, physical therapist, strength and conditioning specialists, hand surgeon, neurosurgeon, dentist, sports chiropractor, nutritionist, psychologist, bioengineer/biomechanist, medical specialist, and other paramedical personnel. The athletic trainer is the hub of this team, as he or she usually provides the first medical care that an injured athlete will receive.

How It Looks Today

Today the hallmarks of a good sports medicine physician are availability, compassion, gentleness, honesty, communication, an understanding of athletic activities, and a true love of injury prevention and healing. Parents and patients alike have a right to expect this kind of treatment from any doctor or athletic trainer working with young athletes.

With any sports medicine team, the number one priority is the player; number two is the player's parents—and only then comes the team, coaches, management, owners, and others. Protecting and preserving a young athlete's safety absolutely must come before big games, league records, championships, scholarships, or anything else that might be tempting to pursue at the cost of the child or teen's health. Parents should feel empowered to speak up and have an active role in their child's care; parents at *all* levels should demand that their young athlete have the availability of a certified athletic trainer. The shared goal of the athlete and the treatment team alike should be the safest way to maximize and prolong a young athlete's career.

Youth sports injuries have reached a crisis point. Immature bones, growing tendons and ligaments, and developing muscles all present a higher risk for injury than many parents and coaches realize. Almost 40 percent of all sports injuries seen in emergency rooms are for children under the age of fourteen. Each year, the number of middle school– and high school–aged students hospitalized for activity-related health concerns also rises. Overuse is the cause of nearly half of all adolescent sports injuries. This disturbing trend must—and can—be stopped through greater awareness, better preparedness, and more thorough education on the issue. Many of these injuries are preventable, yet many teams do not require children to wear the same protective gear or take the same precautions at practices as they do in games.

The goal of modern sports medicine is to make an important shift from treatment to prevention. Although physicians have always advocated injury avoidance, there is a new emphasis on not only how *not* to get injured but also on how to develop stronger, healthier, and more efficient techniques for practicing and competing. In other words, the focus is not simply what to do in order to avoid consequences but also the proactive steps toward reaping greater rewards. Every parent, child, and coach can take positive steps to help build healthy practice habits that will develop the athlete's potential in a way that will maximize the natural talent while developing new skills—and doing so in a way that preserves the child's body for competing at the next level.

Let's be honest: College scholarships and professional contracts are an attractive and exciting part of the business of sports. For older teens, especially, this may be the ultimate goal of many years of hard work and discipline—and who can blame them? Who wouldn't want to have a shot at making a living doing what they love? But when I see a sixteen-year-old on my operating table whose throwing shoulder is as torn up as a forty-six-year-old man's, my heart just breaks because I know that the chances of that young person getting to see his or her dreams come to fruition is highly unlikely—and not because he didn't work hard enough, but because he worked *too* hard (or was pushed too hard) to develop his talent.

The good news is that sports medicine continues to advance. We are at the genesis of radical advancements in the treatment of orthopedic and sports injuries, which I discuss in chapter 35, "The Future of Sports Medicine." Just as the introduction of the arthroscope was a transformational event for sports medicine in the 1970s and 1980s, we are again on the cusp of several new and exciting breakthroughs that are already changing the prognosis of many athletic injuries!

Even so, I think it is essential to point out that the old adage is true: an ounce of prevention really is worth a pound of cure. As logic should tell us, an uninjured joint is always superior to a surgically repaired one. Yet many young athletes are being pushed to a point where their bodies are wearing out far faster than they should be.

Given all the lessons we teach our children about putting what's best for the team above personal performance, it seems counterintuitive that, when it comes to one's health, good sportsmanship means looking out for number one. But that is exactly what needs to happen. Sometimes coaches and managers are too focused on winning to recognize when a player needs to be taken out of the rotation to rest or heal for a few days. Similarly, the most talented athletes are usually competitive by nature and are reluctant to tell their coaches when they need to come out of the game. But an athlete needs to know when further competition will cause more than just discomfort and actually pose a danger to his or her health. That is when a sports medicine team becomes an indispensable part of an athlete's protection.

These professional physicians and trainers are well schooled in how to recognize signs of overuse injuries, concussions, stress fractures, dehydration, or any other of the myriad threats to an athlete's overall health that the coach or player may not even be aware of. Thus, a consultation with an ethical and committed sports medicine practitioner—even just a quick exam on the sidelines or in the dugout—can be a key component in guarding against serious injuries. With this said, an athletic trainer should be present and available in all of our public schools across the country.

STOP Program

In 2005 the American Orthopaedic Society for Sports Medicine established guidelines for selecting team medical coverage. The AOSSM recognizes that many physicians, medical organizations, and teams are committed to maintaining the high standards long established by the medical profession. The selection of team medical staff should be based *not* on financial incentives offered by the physician or his or her institution but on quality of care. The team should fully disclose any sponsorship, advertising, or financial arrangements that the medical staff or its institution has made with the team. The team and medical staff should ensure appropriate communication (within legal limits) with players, other medical providers, and management. Unfortunately, there isn't always a trained sports medicine professional present at youth sports practices or games.

In 2009 the STOP Sports Injuries Campaign was one of the initiatives I helped put into place as part of the AOSSM's core message. Everyone can learn the basics of a healthy pursuit of sports, and everyone has a responsibility to do so. All of the sports medicine disciplines agreed that the time was right to make a major impact on prevention. STOP focuses on the traumatic injuries and overuse injuries associated with more than twenty different youth sports, and promotes better choices for maximized performance.

The Council of Champions is a group of famous figures from the sports and business worlds who share STOP's goals and who work with the steering committee (made up of a number of experienced and well-respected sports medicine physicians) to promote, influence, fund, and stimulate the goals of the STOP program. Council members include John Smoltz, Sam Bradford, Tom Brady, Jack Nicklaus, Brett Favre, Shaquille O'Neal, and Jim Justice, among some thirty others.

Individual Responsibilities

The first step that parents can take to protect their child's athletic future is to take the initiative and responsibility of ensuring that the right safeguards are in place, cooperating with professional medical recommendations, and understanding the role that each party plays in protecting and promoting the young athlete. Many parents have no real sense of the health and injury risk factors associated with youth sports, and I commend anyone who seeks out ways to educate himself or herself on the matter.

With that said, the responsibilities of a sports medicine team (professional and student athletic trainers, emergency personnel, and/or therapists) include:

1. Educating athletes and their parents on proper safety measures for practices and games.

2. Maintaining safe and clean facilities, and watching for any potential hazards.

3. Ensuring the proper fit and maintenance of personal safety equipment.

4. Sideline and on-field care during competition for any physical injury, ranging from minor to catastrophic.

5. Assessment of an athlete's fitness to return to competition following any injury, such as strains, sprains, heat exhaustion, and so on.

6. Making an official record of an athlete's injuries for future reference by the coach.

7. Implementing a rehabilitation regimen for the player unless or until the individual can be examined by a qualified physician.

A sports medicine physician has specialized responsibilities that include but are not limited to the following:

1. Evaluating an aspiring athlete's fitness to participate in organized sports by conducting an athletic physical that includes the child's medical history.

2. Examining and treating any injury requiring advanced medical attention beyond that offered by the sports medicine team.

3. Providing young athletes and their parents with honest and impartial recommendations on whether the child has healed sufficiently to rejoin competition following any major injury, including concussions and fractures.

Coaches and assistant coaches have their own set of responsibilities to the athletes under their supervision:

1. Carefully organizing and overseeing all practices, games, and other team activities.

2. Learning the best conditioning techniques and implementing them in a manner that challenges but does not harm the athletes.

3. Teaching the rules of proper play and sportsmanship.

4. Recognizing signs of injury, including those caused by overuse or fatigue.

5. Obtaining all required certifications in CPR, first aid, and so on.

6. Putting health and competence guidelines above any other aspects of a sport.

Finally, the athlete (as well as his or her parents) has the following responsibilities:

1. Strive for physical fitness.

2. Inform the coach of any health condition of which he or she should be made aware.

3. Maintain proper protective equipment. (Remember that cost does not always equal effectiveness, however. Check the packaging for recommendations from professional medical or athletic organizations. And keep in mind that the most important factor is proper fit.)

4. Study and follow all league rules.

5. Listen to the direction of the coaches and the sports medicine team.

6. Parents should feel empowered to change the sports system in which their child participates if rules and regulations for safety are not adequate or if they are absent altogether.

Why It Matters

It takes a team effort to protect our child athletes. By acknowledging the shared goals, I am confident that we will see not only a drastic reduction in youth sports injuries but also a dramatic rise in the number of young people who are able to pursue their dreams of competition.

Even those children not seeking to play at more elite levels deserve the most enriching athletic experience possible. Good habits of physical activity set early on can last for life. By encouraging the safest possible techniques, we can help all children gain the proven benefits of involvement with organized sports: physical activity, teamwork, socialization, self-confidence, and good sportsmanship.

Chapter 3
Who I Am

Before we get started with the rest of the book, I think it is important to introduce myself by explaining who I am, where I came from, and how it is that I came to focus on the field of orthopedic surgery and sports medicine.

I have had the privilege of being shaped by a number of amazing men and women who believed in me, encouraged me, and helped me find opportunities that would enrich my mind and grow my talents so that I could become the best doctor possible and provide the best care that I could.

Planting the Seed

In some ways, I think I was destined to become a doctor; if it hadn't been something I was naturally interested in, my grandfather would have made sure that it was my career path anyway. Some of my earliest memories are of sitting on my grandfather's lap as we sat on the porch of his farm in north Louisiana, listening to him talk about natural medicines and herbal remedies, and hearing him whisper "You're going to be a doctor someday" with as much pride as if I were already holding my medical school diploma in my chubby little hand. He was a farmer by trade and understood a thing or two about the importance of planting seeds; I think that's exactly what he was doing with me. And so, from childhood, I have always had a sense of the importance of developing young people into the best individuals they can be.

My grandfather, James Nolen, was a remarkable man married to a remarkable woman. He had almost no formal education, but he'd dreamed of becoming a doctor himself. Though he never attended school beyond the first grade in the little rural schoolhouse a dozen miles from his family's farm, he became a kind of country doctor for everyone nearby. He made different salves and ointments for all manner of sores and sicknesses. My grandmother, by comparison, was college educated, which was certainly rare for women in her day. She graduated with a teaching degree from what is now Northwestern State University in Natchitoches, Louisiana. Since she had a knack for numbers, my grandmother ended up keeping all of the books for the farm and handling the accounting for the rest of the family businesses, too.

I was fortunate enough to spend a lot of time around my grandparents when I was young, on account of the fact that my father left to fight in World War II right after I was born, so my mother, sister, and I moved out to the farm for the duration of the war. That gave my grandfather ample opportunity for the first three or four years of my life to talk to me about medicine and give me the nickname "Young Doctor."

It seemed to me to be the most fascinating thing in the world: to learn how the body worked and to help people feel better. And so, from as early as I could remember, I had my sights set on the medical profession. By the time I reached high school, it was the focus of all of my academic energy; my senior English thesis in high school was on plastic surgery, and I can assure you that I was the only kid in Homer, Louisiana, who was that excited about the subject.

My other main interest, however, was sports. If I wasn't trying to read up on the latest advances in medicine, I was involved in a variety of athletics. My father, who had played football at the same college from which my grandmother had graduated, was a real sports nut. He got a tremendous amount of joy in helping out however he was needed and became the unofficial assistant coach/cook/bottle washer for all of the Homer High School sports teams, a feisty bunch of athletes nicknamed, at that time, the Homer Hornmen. We were a small school, so just about everyone participated in just about every sport available, and our football team became a tiny but tenacious powerhouse. My dad was always there, cheering us on at every game. It was wonderful to see him so involved in such a positive way with our teams.

Even more than football, however, I excelled at track and field. In fact, I received a scholarship to Louisiana State University for pole-vaulting. My dad used to drive the three hundred miles from Homer, in the northern part of the state, all the way down to Baton Rouge just to watch me practice and to encourage me. He was never pushy about my practice habits, just supportive and excited about my talent.

Because of my love of medicine and my love of sports, I desperately wanted to bring the two together professionally. I assumed that I would become a team physician for a college somewhere, which meant that I should try for an orthopedic surgical residency as my specialty in medical school; the term *sports medicine* was not yet widely in use. And med school came a little sooner than I had anticipated. My father died suddenly at the end of my sophomore year at LSU. I vaulted for one more year and won the indoor and outdoor pole-vault championships, but my heart wasn't in it in the same way after losing my biggest fan. I decided to forego my senior year and head straight to LSU Medical School in New Orleans, where I had earned a full legislative grant. Looking back now, I kind of regret having skipped my last year as an undergraduate, but I was eager to get on with my life. I thought I might compete as an "unattached" athlete (meaning that I was still eligible but not part of an undergraduate team) while in med school, but the reality of the workload and new pursuits crowded that out. For this reason, I have always understood how a young athlete feels about having to cut his or her athletic career short, and how that athlete will often try to find a reason to compete despite pain or stress. I'd find new outlets for my competitive bug, but my days as a pole-vaulter were over. It was time to focus on medicine.

Dr. James R. Andrews

Exploring the Field

I had some fascinating times and met some incredible people in medical school, but the most instrumental part of setting my career path came during my residency at Tulane University. We had what were called sound-slide presentations, where we would examine slides that the American Academy of Orthopaedic Surgeons would put out on various subjects with accompanying narration and explanation. The presentation that really captured my attention more than any others was an hour-long sound-slide study on acute knee ligament injuries in football players presented by Dr. Jack C. Hughston from Columbus, Georgia. One slide had a photo of Dr. Hughston standing by a sign that said "Welcome to the City of Auburn," and he had his foxhounds standing beside him. He was introduced as the team physician for Auburn University, and he absolutely became my idol. I began to read everything I could by him and about him and desperately wanted to become his protégé.

I learned that Dr. Hughston, who founded the Hughston Clinic in 1949, was one of the fathers of sports medicine in the United States and was well respected not only in the Southeast but also across the nation and around the world. He represented to me everything I wanted to do with my medical practice. In addition to helping athletes recover after injuries, he was helping in the education and care of amateur athletes at large universities and small high schools. On that last point, he reminded me of my grandfather, in that he was offering a service to people in rural communities that were often overlooked and underserved. In fact, before Dr. Hughston, there was virtually no medical coverage at high school games. He single-handedly helped to bring about that change.

By my second year of residency, I had decided that I would reach out to Dr. Hughston to see if I could get to know him better and perhaps visit him. He invited me immediately, so after my work was completed on Friday, I drove the eight hours from New Orleans to the Hughston Clinic in Columbus, Georgia, to shadow him for the weekend: from his Friday-night high school games, to his Saturday-morning knee surgeries, to his Saturday-afternoon college football games. Sunday afternoon I drove back to Louisiana in time for my shift, but I was absolutely hooked after that first weekend.

I asked Dr. Hughston if it might be possible for me to spend some time with him during my residency. He was just starting up what we called "apprenticeships" for residents and postgraduate residents to work in his practice to learn about sports medicine. Dr. Hughston was a tremendously enthusiastic man, and he loved to see that same enthusiasm in other people, so he did me one better than just lining up a short-term apprenticeship. He actually called my chief at Tulane, Dr. Jack Wickstrom, to formally invite me to study sports medicine in Columbus and to pitch the idea of spending my entire third year of residency working the games and in his sports medicine clinic. I don't know what Dr. Hughston said or how he did it, but for some reason, Dr. Wickstrom agreed. I left Charity Hospital in New Orleans, and instead of doing my third year with an emphasis on trauma patients, as is usually the case, I went to work with Dr. Hughston as a fellow for that entire next year.

Growing Time

Under Dr. Hughston's guidance, I finished my residency and then got a fellowship with Dr. Frank McCue III, the team physician for the University of Virginia. This was a particularly good opportunity because Dr. McCue was an expert on upper extremity surgery, which I wanted to learn about because I could see how that would be important for athletes in a number of sports, including baseball and golf. Dr. McCue was a brilliant man and the epitome of everything that a team physician should be in terms of both his tremendous medical knowledge as well as his concern for the players' long-term health. He had an air of professionalism about him that instilled a sense of calm and confidence in whomever he was treating. As a young doctor studying his techniques, I saw what kind of team physician I hoped to become one day.

In 1972, following my study with Dr. McCue, Dr. Hughston

reached out to Professor Albert Trillat, who was the father of modern knee surgery in Europe and the chief of orthopedics at the University of Lyon in France. I was invited for a fellowship that lasted roughly eight months and allowed me to learn more about the European techniques in knee surgery. It was a fascinating and eye-opening experience to see how the same injuries could be treated in slightly different ways. Professor Trillat is the man who taught me a truism I have seen proven over and over in my own career: "The only results that I remember are my bad ones." That may seem like a rather glum perspective, but, really, it is very helpful for a surgeon to learn from his or her mistakes.

All these mentors molded my medical philosophy in real and important ways, and their patience, wisdom, and guidance are responsible for any successes I have had in my career.

Upon my return to the States, I began practicing with Dr. Hughston in January 1973. He was still taking care of Auburn University, but one of the things he stressed to me was that availability and communication are the two key components in being a successful sports medicine physician. He encouraged me to not just hang around with him at Auburn but also spread our energy and our resources to smaller colleges. He had nudged me in this direction when I was still a resident with him in 1969, and we worked with Troy State College (now Troy University) in Troy, Alabama. Now, in addition to Troy, I branched out to many smaller colleges and universities, including Tuskegee, Livingston (now the University of West Alabama), North Alabama, Jacksonville State, Grambling, and several others with football teams.

I soon came to realize that while the injury rates at all schools were similar, the smaller schools often lacked medical personnel to cover their athletic events. Wasn't the health of those athletes every bit as important as the athletes at Division I schools? This became a very passionate issue for me, and so I began a pattern of crazy Saturdays that would become one of the standard practices of my career, in some form or another, to this day.

Each Saturday, I would attend the Auburn game with Dr. Hughston and stay as long as I could. Then I would board a small airplane (I had a Cessna 182 in those days) and would fly to each of the smaller schools, from game to game, to see if anyone needed immediate care. During the week, I would offer clinics at those schools, as well as an outreach program for college athletes and high school students in the surrounding areas—some of which were out in the boondocks in rural Alabama. At the time, no other doctors offered that kind of medical treatment, so we weren't competing with anyone locally, and it was a great opportunity to develop our relationships with some of those communities and young athletes. It was all part of Dr. Hughston's tremendous vision that we were able to make this happen. While my ultimate goal was still to be the team physician for a Division I school, I found myself fostering a deep loyalty to the smaller schools I worked with during that time, and I really cut my teeth at Troy University in particular.

A few years later, I finally tried my hand as the lead physician for a major university sports program, at the University of Kentucky. I served in that capacity for several years before moving down to Birmingham in 1986, but I also continued to assist Dr. Hughston and Kenny Howard, head athletic trainer at Auburn. I was extremely fortunate at Kentucky to serve under two great head coaches: football coach Jerry Claiborne and basketball coach Joe B. Hall. In 1992, Dr. Hughston was preparing to retire and Terry Bowden replaced Pat Dye as head football coach at Auburn. Coach Bowden hired me as Dr. Hughston's successor. It was thrilling to follow so closely in my mentor's footsteps, and working as the team physician for both Auburn and the University of Alabama remains one of my proudest accomplishments. (Since taking over as the medical director for Auburn, I must mention that I have been fortunate enough to have Dr. Mike Goodlett as my eyes and ears full-time at Auburn as the head team physician.) It has certainly been a challenge at times, working for the two largest universities in the state (and great athletic rivals) simultaneously, but it has also been tremendously rewarding—especially getting to be part of the National Championship program two years in a row. Auburn won the 2010 title, and Alabama captured it in 2011. Some people just shake their heads when they find out that I have a relationship with Auburn *and* Alabama, but for me it's an honor to ensure the health and well-being of so many athletes in our state.

Dr. James R. Andrews

My Mentor

Dr. Jack C. Hughston has had the most profound influence on me of anyone I studied under. He was the kind of person who knew how to get the last bit of effort out of those around him. Your best was never good enough if he knew you had more to give. I don't mean that in a negative way; he never made you feel like a failure, but he was going to work you to the bone—and you'd do it happily because you respected him so much! For a personality type like mine, which is always eager to please and very concerned with making people happy, this kind of relationship with my mentor absolutely wore me out, but it made me a heck of a better doctor in the process! Every time I reached a point where I thought he'd be happy, Dr. Hughston would push me to go even further. Yet he never expected anyone to do anything that he wouldn't do. He always got up earlier, worked later, and got more accomplished than everyone under him who was trying to keep up.

As you can see, nobody could ever match Dr. Hughston's ability to motivate people. His burning desire to succeed rubbed off on all the people who worked around him.

For example, Dr. Hughston had a favorite saying: "The work is never done until the paperwork is completed." If you did not finish your paperwork, whatever you'd done in the operating room did not count. He wanted to make sure that every doctor under his supervision saw the job through to the very end. If you slacked off in one part of a patient's care, who was to say you wouldn't slack off elsewhere, too? But even more than that, paperwork ensured that we could learn from each and every patient. He was insistent about the importance of documentation—that was his big word. You have to *document* everything that you do so that you know if you are doing it right.

Dr. Hughston also stressed the importance of research. In fact, he was the founder of some of the scientific principles that we all live by in modern sports medicine, as well as the founder-editor of the *American Journal of Sports Medicine*. In 1972, when the American Orthopaedic Society of Sports Medicine was established, he was also instrumental in developing its vision and platform. Sometimes he would wake up in the middle of the night and start working furiously on charts or a scientific paper. It wasn't uncommon to find him writing a chapter for a book he was researching at four o'clock in the morning, having gone to bed at midnight. When we would make hospital rounds early in the morning, Dr. Hughston wanted all the fellows to join him—but he would always beat you there. If he said that we would make rounds at six o'clock, we'd all assemble at six only to discover that he had been making rounds already since five thirty. The next day, we would get there at five thirty, and he would have been making rounds at five. We could never ever outdo him or outmaneuver him. Those were just the games he played to keep us motivated.

The other thing that Dr. Hughston was so good at was record keeping. He used to make drawings of *where* a patient's ligaments were injured, so that later he could write up a scientific paper knowing exactly what the injury was and what parts of the knee were actually injured. Even before computers, Dr. Hughston was the consummate record keeper. He never got rid of any of his old records, just in case he needed to reference an old chart or revisit a certain case. At the first office that we had in Columbus, Georgia, it seemed as if the entire tiny space was taken up by paperwork. In fact, there was one patient we saw from time to time whose file seemed to be ten feet thick. But if you looked closely, you realized that the file was labeled "Patient 1," and it was the first person he had ever seen in his clinic from when he first went into practice. It was amazing to me that he still had that very first patient's chart for documentation.

Dr. Hughston also used to check your dictations to see if you were doing them right, and he would mark them up with his ever-present red ballpoint pen if you weren't. He was a perfectionist, but he did it because it mattered. He wanted to make sure that every doctor working with him was providing the best possible care for every last patient.

Usually seen wearing his trademark bow tie, Dr. Hughston modeled for me every item in my patient philosophy, which I will talk about below. For that, I am forever indebted to him. He taught those of us studying under him not only how to be good doctors but also how to talk to athletes.

He always stressed that a major part of being a physician was in how you presented yourself and how patients perceived you. Heaven forbid that you ever looked less than respectable when dealing with patients! That was a mistake you made only once in front of Dr. Hughston. It was the little things like that, he explained, that made all the difference in giving athletes confidence in our expertise. As a result, we always wore a coat and tie to work, and to this day, you won't see me around the hospital or the clinic in anything else. He also had the same dress code when we covered high school and college football games. If you will notice on the sidelines, most of the sports medicine doctors dress up like coaches. That's normal (and required) for NFL team doctors, but even when I am on the sidelines for Auburn or Alabama, I'm wearing a coat and tie. Now, I can't pull off a bow tie like Dr. Hughston used to wear, but I do dress up the way a respected physician should.

The Alabama native, who passed away in 2004 at the age of eighty-seven, also taught me about how important it was to cultivate good relationships with trainers, coaches, and athletes alike. Dr. Hughston taught me to respect trainers and therapists as equals and to support them in everything that we do because, really, we share the same goal. He was a major supporter of the National Athletic Trainers' Association and the American Physical Therapy Association, and often spoke at their conventions as well as invited them to our sports medicine meetings. It was through these interactions that I had the chance to first meet some of the most outstanding trainers with whom I have ever had the pleasure to work.

Dr. Hughston's ability to communicate was the reason that athletes flocked to him. He understood the sports they played. He was able to talk to them in a way that earned their trust and convinced them to listen. He got down to their level. That was the most important aspect of his being on the sidelines with them instead of just waiting in his office Monday morning to see the players hobble in for treatment. He was there when they got hurt; he saw what happened. He taught us that the evaluation on the field and management of on-the-field injuries were the most important aspects of providing early treatment.

Dr. Hughston was big on rehabilitation, too. He was probably as well known for his rehabilitation regimens of athletic injuries as he was for his surgical interventions. He always had top specialists in sports injury rehabilitation working with him. Those individuals were Kenny Howard, head athletic trainer for Auburn, and George McCluskey, a registered physical therapist in charge of all the rehabilitation treatments for Auburn players. McCluskey had his own physical therapy clinic adjacent to Dr. Hughston's. I have always modeled that relationship by having an exceptionally talented team of rehabilitation specialists and athletic trainers work with me wherever I have been.

And in all of this, he never asked for any recognition or sought out press for the ways in which he was revolutionizing the field. In fact, he thought that if you were out trying to market yourself, you were making a big mistake, and if accolades were your main motivation, you were not going to be a truly good doctor.

Really, everything I have done to be successful in sports medicine is just a culmination of all the things that I learned from Dr. Hughston. I merely added my own personality and flavor to the way I do things, but I owe everything to him and his unrelenting pursuit of the finest patient care.

My Philosophy

Today, as I am now in my fifth decade of practicing medicine, I live and breathe by the personal philosophy I developed during all those years of training and experience.

The rules by which I conduct myself and my practice are, I believe, the most important guidelines for effective care and successful treatment. I would urge any athlete seeking medical care to be aware of these standards and to seek out a doctor who approaches patient care similarly. In no way am I implying, of course, that a doctor who does not share the same philosophy cannot be a good doctor, but I do think that it is essential for patients to have a sense of what their rights are and what they should expect from their doctors.

The following list is posted openly in all of my clinics:

Patient Philosophy

1. *The patient is always right.* So often doctors treat what they assume the problem is rather than what the patient is really telling them. The patient has a right to describe his or her symptoms as they exist rather than as the treating physician assumes they are. If the patient is not trusted to know his or her own pain, treatment becomes nearly impossible.

2. *Make the patient feel he was treated properly by his previous physician.* I always cringe when I hear someone say that he went for a second opinion and the doctor discounted everything that the first doctor did. This can be extremely damaging to a patient's sense of well-being. It is highly doubtful that the previous physician did absolutely nothing helpful or well; the new doctor on the case needs to bear that in mind and assure the patient that progress has been made, even if he or she plans on proceeding in a different direction treatment-wise.

3. *Do not say anything negative about another physician or another person, for that matter.* This is basically the same advice I received from my mother: "If you can't say something nice about someone, don't say anything at all." That holds true in our personal lives as well as professionally.

4. *Always be open-minded.* It is extremely important for practicing physicians to be willing to learn new things, study new discoveries and developments in the field, and be conscious of the fact that no matter how much we have read, seen, and worked—we do not know everything!

5. *Listen to the patient.* This ties in with rule number one but goes further. Doctors need to listen to the patient to learn the symptoms and complaints so that they can diagnose the problem. But just as important, a doctor needs to get to know the patient and his or her habits. Especially in a field like sports medicine, this is key to preventing future injuries. Learn the patient's practice

schedule and talk to her about her habits. All of these things make a huge difference in the care you are able to offer. Plus, when patients feel that their doctor is really listening to them, it gives them confidence in the treatment regimen as well, which means they will be more likely to follow it.

6. *Do not be the first person to make the "big statement."* This was something that Dr. Hughston stressed a great deal. The treating physician should not be the first one to make a dramatic statement such as, "It looks like your playing days are over." Maybe the injury is so catastrophic that it is highly doubtful that the athlete will ever be able to recapture his or her former glory. However, we need to wait for the patient to ask the question before we offer our opinion. This does two things: It allows the patient to wrap his or her head around the situation and warm up to it in degrees, and it also keeps the doctor from becoming too "God-like" in everyone's eyes (including his or her own!).

7. *Attitude, responsibility, knowledge, desire, and availability are always necessary to be successful.* This is self-explanatory, and it is true for every profession. These five attributes affect the way we approach every job and will determine our success or failure. It's that simple.

8. *One must always be able to "read the patient."* Interpersonal skills are essential to how we interact with patients. This doesn't just mean that doctors should have a good bedside manner (although that helps, of course), but we must also be able to evaluate the patient to see if there are any missing "clues" for an accurate diagnosis, effective treatment, and a healthier future. And a physician should always communicate with the patient at his or her level.

9. *The physician must be confident about his diagnosis and surgical skills.* His confidence is reflected back and perceived by the patient. If a patient does not feel confident in a physician's skill set, that can greatly hamper the healing process. Doctors must present themselves with confidence (but not arrogance), so as to put the patient

at ease. And what is the best way to generate confidence? To actually possess the knowledge, skills, and understanding necessary to complete the task you're given.

I hope that this short introduction has allowed you to get a better sense of who I am, my perspectives on the field of sports medicine, and how I came to hold those views. I have been blessed with a series of tremendous opportunities and incredible experiences, but I came from humble beginnings and have always tried to keep that in mind. Every day, I remind myself what a great privilege it is to get to do what I love. No, I am not curing cancer or eradicating childhood hunger or anything of the sort, but I am entrusted with helping people improve their quality of life—and, in many cases, their dreams.

As much as I love my job, however, I wish it were unnecessary. I wish that no one ever ended up on my operating table because of a severe injury. Unfortunately, we all know that isn't reality. But I do hope that this book will help to greatly reduce the number of patients in need of extreme medical intervention and will provide young athletes with a better shot at chasing their dreams, just as I was able to chase mine.

Chapter 4
The Doctor Recommends

It was George Bernard Shaw who quipped famously, "Youth is wasted on the young." The older I get, the truer that statement seems to be. Now that I'm in the twilight of my career, after a lifetime of studying and treating injuries in teenagers and adults, I can see that the feeling of invincibility that comes with youth is nearly universal. I certainly know that I believed James Andrews was absolutely unstoppable when I was in my twenties and thirties—but now, my aches and pains are like a scrapbook of all of my crazy moments, my daredevil stunts, and the times I decided just to "rub some dirt on it" when I took a big hit in football or a hard fall in pole-vaulting.

I firmly believe that the human body is the most fascinating and interesting machine ever created. But the truth is that the human body, like any machine, wears out with time. It's hard to believe that when you're young and fit and your body has never failed you—or has always been able to quickly repair itself after it did. As anyone with a few more decades under his or her belt will tell you, though, that feeling of being utterly unstoppable is an illusion. In time it will catch up to you, and all those aches and pains and creaks and cracks that you always thought were someone else's problem will become your own. Sometimes it's a creeping realization; sometimes the aging process seems to happen almost overnight. Whatever the case, the day will come when the young athlete is no longer young and starts to pay the wages of all the years of pushing his or her body to the extreme. In fact, any traumatic injury suffered in childhood exponentially increases the chance for arthritis in middle age or old age. That's just the way it goes. Everything is cumulative—you'll have to face the music at some point or another.

So what is the solution? To never set foot outside? To never strap on a helmet? To never pick up a racket? Quite the opposite. Lifestyle choices made in youth are cumulative as well. For example, carrying extra weight—even just putting on a few pounds a year—adds up over a lifetime. Think about it: A young man who weighs a healthy 150 pounds at age twenty and gains just 5 pounds a year will have *doubled* his weight by the age of fifty to tip the scale at 300 pounds! It doesn't take a doctor to recognize the cardiovascular risks and heightened odds of developing diabetes that accompany such a substantial weight gain. Of course, children and teens should expect to see their weight increase as they grow, their bodies develop into adult forms, and their muscle mass increases. But if a youngster gets used to exceeding a healthy weight at age fifteen, chances are that he or she will continue to carry extra pounds through adulthood, adding a little more each year.

I see it all the time. People work their entire lives for retirement, when they finally have the time, money, and freedom to pursue their interests or to travel the world. However, if they did not make wise choices concerning their bodies when they were young, they may not have the health to enjoy retirement once they reach it. Believe me, I know. A few years ago, I had to undergo heart surgery, and it really shook me up to realize that I was not invincible. I started thinking back to all the choices I'd made regarding diet, exercise, habits, hobbies—and it made me realize that there were a lot of things that I would have done differently if I'd really stopped to think about the lingering health effects of those decisions.

So how do parents protect their active children and motivate the ones who are prone to be more sedentary? The simplest answer for both is "gradual steps." Young athletes who are excited to get back on the field or the court or into the pool can endanger themselves by beginning their training too aggressively at first, tearing muscles or overusing joints that have not been conditioned sufficiently. Coaches and parents alike need to encourage a child's enthusiasm for a sport while also making sure that safeguards are in place so that an injury doesn't end a season before it even begins.

For several years I was involved in trying to get two weeks of spring training added to the schedule for youth baseball teams in the hopes of easing youngsters into the routine of practice and conditioning. The intention was for each team to have a little bit longer to ramp up their activity. What happened instead was that many coaches simply seized upon that extra time to start playing their athletes hard for an additional two weeks. Especially for athletes who are highly motivated and want to give their all at every practice, this kind of intensive training puts them at a much higher risk for overuse injuries because the body simply is not prepared to handle what it's being asked to do.

Many young athletes will not speak up because they don't want to get pulled from a game, let down their teammates, or disappoint a parent. Sometimes an athlete will confide in one parent but not the other about a potential injury. Parents and coaches need to be attuned to the young people under their care and watch for warning signs. It's one thing to feel some soreness in the muscles a day or two after a workout—that means they are being stretched and developed. But it's another thing entirely when the muscles are so sore that they limit normal movement. Always remember: The goal is to be *better* each day, not worse.

On the other hand, children and teens who are not athletically inclined will need extra encouragement to exercise or get involved in a sport. The challenge in this situation is determining the difference between the "good" soreness of a workout routine and the "bad" soreness that results from an injury. Obviously, a child who is used to playing nothing more than video games is probably going to feel a stitch in the side and burning lungs when trying to run a mile for the first time. How can coaches and parents distinguish when to encourage the child to keep going and when to take those complaints seriously and stop the training? Again, the key is to focus on gradual conditioning. Don't expect a youngster to be able to run a seven-minute mile on the first day of training. Start with something simpler. For example, suggest that the child alternate between walking and jogging each lap. And don't push beyond an hour of activity at first. Try one day on and one day off for an exercise schedule. Build up to two days on, one day off; and then three days on, two days off—until you reach the standard five-days-on, two-days-off schedule that most high school athletes follow. This helps the child or teen gain a sense of accomplishment. If a child is not enjoying a sport, try a different activity, such as recreational cycling or martial arts. At least in the earliest stages, these are much lower impact than most youth sports and can be great gateway activities to help establish a basic level of fitness. The point is that some kind of physical exertion is necessary for healthy living. Children and teens need to have some kind of activity to serve as an outlet, a means of positive social interaction, a supervised way to stay out of trouble, and a means of fending off later health challenges.

That being said, parents should never brush off a child's complaints about pain. Even if he or she is probably just feeling the body's natural response to new activity (or even if the parent suspects strongly that the child is just whining), they should never assume that nothing is wrong. Talk to your youngster about the nature of the discomfort. Try to detect any patterns or links between the pain and certain types of movement to see if activity should be adapted to allow for healing. Encourage him or her to talk to the school nurse or the team's athletic trainer. Before introducing any sport, take your child to the pediatrician for a physical exam. (This is required by most school leagues anyway.) Don't turn a blind eye to the complaint; sometimes real issues do exist that were previously undetected or have developed over time.

Parents need to be involved and need to listen to their children. For most young athletes, Mom and Dad are their first line of support and most effective advocates. Invest yourself in your child's overall health and work to protect it, whether it is getting him active in the first place or looking out for her long-term potential by preventing overuse or traumatic injuries today. If we put our children's safety first, chances are that they will be able to enjoy a longer time pursuing the sport that they love. The more steps we can take to keep our children healthy when they are young, the greater chance their bodies will serve them well through adulthood and into old age.

This isn't an easy lesson to teach to kids. After all, if they feel great all the time, why should they believe that they ever won't? Would you have believed at sixteen that you might ever have stiffness in your knees or not be able to move your shoulders like you used to? The aging process is unimaginable to most kids, just as it was to us. Far more effective than simply preaching at kids is to model positive behavior ourselves. A child is more likely to imitate the choices made in his or her own home; for example, seeing parents pursuing healthy lifestyles in terms of physical fitness, diet, protective equipment in sports, proper stretching and warm-ups, strength conditioning, and any of the other preventative measures one can take to keep the body in good shape or to get in shape.

It's our responsibility to protect our kids. Let's speak up for them, cheer them on, and make the kinds of choices in our own lives that will empower them to make good choices too. It's about preserving the future for each kid, whether he or she will go on to become a professional athlete, a college star, or just a healthy adult well equipped to enjoy a happy and fulfilling life.

Part 2

A Handbook of Youth Sports Injuries

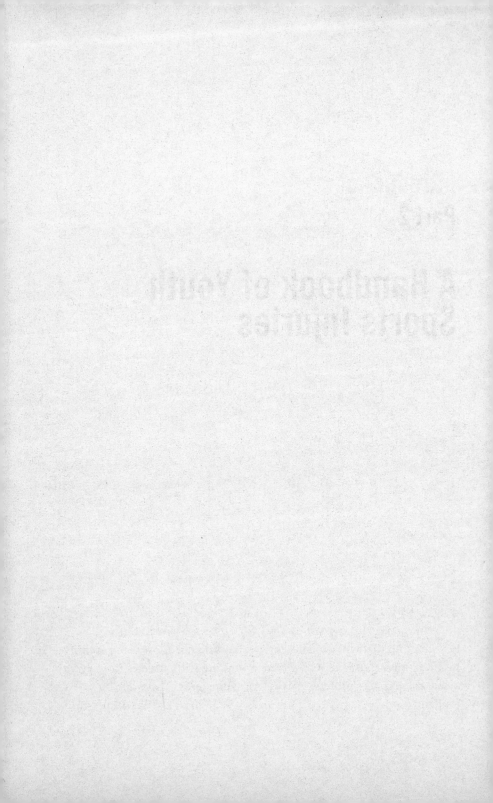

Introduction

It's a daunting task to try to document every possible health risk in every single popular youth sport. For example, although I discuss running, I do not address the various potential injuries associated with field events such as discus, javelin, or triple jump—and I was a pole-vaulter myself! There are just too many different activities to highlight. What I have tried to do is to cover as broad a range of sports as possible: from endurance sports, to aquatic sports, to ice sports, to court sports, and beyond, not to mention all the different genres of dance and martial arts. My hope is that the following chapters contain enough helpful information and guidance regarding the most common types of sports-related injuries, the treatment options available, and (better yet) steps for avoiding them.

Some chapters are much shorter than others, due to the nature of the injuries discussed. It doesn't mean that these activities are less significant or that participants face less risk of injury. It simply means I have not personally seen or treated as many cases from which I can make specific prevention guidelines based on my own experience. And readers should keep in mind that while medical privacy laws do not allow me to identify specific individuals, I have experience working with athletes from every one of these sports: professionals as well as amateurs. I have done my best to identify which activities tend to attract the most participants, which ones I can speak on with authority, and which injuries tend to plague those athletes so that parents, players, coaches, grandparents, and anyone else who is interested and concerned about the issue will have a starting point for awareness and further action.

Of course, there is always the challenge of repetition; I did not want to repeat the exact same information every single time a certain risk is mentioned. Because concussions are so foundational, I have devoted a chapter to them, as well as the importance of having an emergency action plan (chapter 31). Other injuries, such as ACL tears, for example, are common in just about every "cutting" sport—that is, one that employs rapid movement and sudden changes of direction—so I made sure to outline the symptoms in each potential scenario. But since ACL tears are repairable only by surgery, which will require a physician's diagnosis, I did not go into great detail as to how the condition should be treated on the field. I will say that in an effort to combat the rise of ACL injuries among young athletes (especially young women), some schools now offer classes in proper jumping and landing form in the so-called athletic posture: knees bent, feet apart. I will discuss more about these programs below.

That is why I would encourage readers to avoid the temptation to read only the one or two chapters applicable to your child's sport or activity, and to at least peruse the other chapters as well. Familiarize yourself with the risks and treatment recommendations. Maybe they will come in handy for your own child's training, or maybe they will just help you to understand the bigger picture of injury prevention in youth sports. Either way, there is something to be gained. My greatest concern is that most parents are not fully aware of the risk of injury their child faces in a particular sport. I hope that this book will help change that.

The Female Athlete Triad

I also believe that it is important to take a moment to discuss the significance of the "female athlete triad" and the risks that it poses to all young women who compete in sports, but especially those whose weight can affect their competitive status by placing them in different weight classes (such as martial arts) or whose body shape may affect their role on the team or within the perceived "norms" of the activity (such as with cheerleading, dance, gymnastics, and figure skating). But the truth is that social pressure as well as personal drive can lead any young female athlete to develop issues associated with the triad.

The term *female athlete triad* pertains to three conditions that pose unique health risks for young women who are very physically active and pursue sports aggressively: eating disorders, amenorrhea, and osteoporosis. Sometimes the athlete is affected by all three; sometimes only one or two of the branches affect her. Whatever the case, these disorders are serious and can have long-term implications for a young woman's physical health, emotional strength, and overall well-being, and they tend to progress from one condition to the next.

Eating Disorders

In an effort to bolster her athletic performance by altering her body's muscle-to-fat ratio, a female athlete may change her eating habits. This is not simply a move to a healthier diet, however; some young women may suddenly cut out all types of a certain food that they perceive as being too fattening or otherwise detrimental to their health, even if the food isn't "bad" at all. Parents should pay close attention to what, when, and how their daughter eats. If a sudden change in quantity or type of food is detected, it is vital that this be discussed to make sure that the choice is a healthy one and not something that she is viewing as a "magic fix" for whatever is bothering her. If she is pinning her hopes of improvement on dietary changes, she is more likely to take them to an extreme, possibly even leading to anorexia nervosa (purposely starving oneself) or bulimia nervosa (binge eating followed by purging through vomiting or consuming laxatives). While these conditions can also affect young men, they are far more predominant among females and can lead to the next part of the triad: amenorrhea.

Amenorrhea

When the female body does not receive sufficient nutrients to keep up with its level of activity, it will often cut back on its manufacture of estrogen, the predominant female hormone and the one that triggers regular menstrual cycles. While it is true that girls who have just begun menstruating may not always have regular cycles, skipped periods for athletes can also indicate unbalanced estrogen levels. There may also be cause for concern if an athletic young woman fails to start her period by the age of fifteen. In some cases, it may simply be that she is a late developer; however, the absence of a period may also be due to a consistently low estrogen level brought about by extreme physical exertion in athletic training. Young women should make a note on their calendars each time they have a period, and whether the flow seems heavier or lighter than usual. This can prove a valuable tool if the cycle seems to suddenly change or stop altogether. One of the very first things a doctor will want to know is the date of the young woman's last period and if the changes have coincided with any changes in behavior, including athletic training, sexual activity, and diet.

Osteoporosis

If amenorrhea continues unchecked, it may lead to the third part of the triad, which is osteoporosis, or a decrease in bone density that can lead to fragility of the bones, malformation, and stunted growth. Again, although this condition can also affect men, it is exponentially more common in women, and young female athletes are especially at risk if they have deprived their bodies of proper nutrition. It is essential that young women have a steady supply of calcium in their diets, as well as healthy levels of other vitamins and minerals required to allow the body to grow and develop normally. Bone density only decreases with age, which greatly heightens the risk for small breaks in the bone known as stress fractures. These breaks, which occur not from a traumatic bone injury but from accumulated stress overload, can cut short even the most promising athletic career. Young women whose bones are not sufficiently developed in their teenage years will face more severe health challenges as they enter adulthood and beyond.

Warning Signs

Parents, grandparents, coaches, and teammates should be on the lookout for red flags such as sudden weight loss or an obsession with weight loss, decreased energy, repeated injuries to the same joint or bone, brittle fingernails and hair, tooth loss or cavities (which, in athletes with bulimia, can be the result of regurgitated stomach acid eroding the enamel), frequent trips to the bathroom following meals, and stress fractures. Although any of these might be a symptom of something else or just part of a young woman's natural body condition, it is important to speak up if you have a concern. Don't be afraid to sit down with the athlete herself and explain what has you worried and why; concerned parents may wish to make an appointment with a dietitian or counselor who specializes in eating disorders to get a better handle on healthy food choices and eating habits. It is better to have an uncomfortable conversation and prevent a tragedy than to have to deal with the aftermath of a deteriorating body later.

If concerned friends and family rally around a young woman who is facing the female athlete triad, she stands a much better chance of making a full recovery. Not only will this support allow her to reach her personal best in a safe manner, but it will also give her a much better chance at a full and healthy future by protecting her body from premature aging, damage, and other potentially life-limiting conditions.

Growing Pains

Many children, especially between the ages of eight and twelve, will often complain of throbbing pain in their legs and arms late in the day or at night. It is quite possible that what they are feeling is not a sports injury at all but the natural response of the muscles to being stretched as the bones lengthen—in other words, growing pains. These sensations usually do not affect joints and are felt more acutely in the larger muscles of the body, such as the calves and the quadriceps. While they are harmless (though sometimes painful), do not dismiss a youngster's complaint as nothing more than growing pains, because you may be overlooking a serious issue. Listen to your child and allow him or her to explain what hurts; pay attention to your child's practice schedule and see if you can detect any patterns or links between complaints of pain and certain activities. Remember that proper precautions can prevent serious injuries, and, as grandmothers the world over love to say, "An ounce of prevention is worth a pound of cure."

ACL Injury Prevention and Performance Enhancement

Despite the wonderfully positive rise in participation in youth sports by young women, there is a negative consequence: Serious knee ligament injuries among female athletes have reached epidemic proportions. This is particularly true in girls' soccer and other cutting sports such as basketball and volleyball. Female athletes have a two- to ten-fold increase for noncontact ACL knee injuries compared to their male counterparts. An estimated 110,000 to 200,000 high school and collegiate female athletes will sustain a serious knee ligament injury annually. These injuries usually require surgical reconstruction followed by extensive rehabilitation. The majority of affected patients lose an entire athletic season, which can lead to a possible loss of scholarship funding. In addition, some injured athletes also suffer lower academic performance and class attendance as a result.

There are several ACL injury prevention programs that have been established around the country. Two of the most notable ones are SportsMetrics, headed by Frank Noyes of the Cincinnati SportsMedicine and Orthopaedic Center in Cincinnati, Ohio; the other one was developed by Bert Mendelbaum of the Santa Monica Orthopaedic and Sports Medicine Group. Dr. Noyes, a well-known leader in knee surgery and a pioneer in the treatment of ACL injuries, started this program to help prevent injuries in both male and female athletes. Dr. Mendelbaum is also a prominent and well-respected sports medicine specialist with an interest in soccer and injury prevention. These programs, among others, provide important training during the summer months for junior high and high school athletes, with the goal of significantly reducing the risk of serious knee ligament injuries and enhancing performance by increasing lower extremity strength and vertical jump heights, and decreasing lower extremity muscular imbalances. Young athletes receive hands-on instruction and training techniques to provide an excellent foundation in sports-specific training by certified instructors in local communities. Currently, there are more than 790 sites across the United States and around the world that provide reciprocal website links to promote the certified clinical sites. Dr. Noyes and SportsMetrics have a course that certifies athletic trainers and clinical sites as well. The aim is to reach as many young athletes as possible. There are other, similar independent courses in other parts of the country that are also excellent. Any interested parent or grandparent should look into what programs are available locally or promote and collaborate on their development if you live in an area without one of these courses.

Magnetic Resonance Imaging (MRI) Scans: Necessary or Not?

While magnetic resonance imaging (MRI) can be a great diagnostic tool, it does not take the place of having a well-qualified sports medicine doctor examine the injury, compile a complete medical history, and order routine X-rays. We hear on the news often that some sports star or another is "awaiting an MRI for diagnosis." Unfortunately, this has led many people to believe that if their child does not receive an MRI, the doctor is not providing the best care possible. This simply is not true. An MRI is not always necessary, nor does it always help to identify the problem any better than more traditional means of diagnosis. Sometimes, as is the case with any medical technology, the images can even be somewhat misleading as to the nature or extent of the injury. I have given second opinions to many young patients who had seen some of the finest sports medicine doctors and orthopedists I know. And the only reason they scheduled a consultation with me was that their parents were upset that the first doctor did not order an MRI. Similarly, I have seen patients decline to start treatment or physical therapy for the same reason. I urge parents to please understand that MRI scans are very expensive procedures that are very often simply not required for making an accurate diagnosis. If you are concerned about the level of care that your child is receiving, of course you should seek out a different provider; if, however, your only concern is the lack of an MRI, I would ask you to please understand that it should not be the first step in a diagnosis.

Much of the information covered in the following chapters can be found on the STOP program website at www.stopsportsinjuries.org. I encourage readers to treat the website as a companion to this book. The more we educate ourselves about the risks facing our children, the more equipped we'll be to set up our kids for a life of physical fitness, camaraderie, goal setting, and everything else that sports have to offer.

Chapter 5
Baseball

It's one of the most coveted positions in all of youth sports: the starting pitcher for the local Little League team. It used to be that some coaches started their top hurler in every game, confident that their star's arm would help cinch one win after the other. And maybe he'd develop his talent to the point of playing in the majors some day.

But all of that has changed, with leagues now protecting their young hurlers, and I count it as one of the greatest accomplishments of my career that I helped to make that happen. Of course, injuries such as sprains and abrasions can occur in any position in baseball; however, without a doubt, the pitcher is the most vulnerable player when it comes to potentially career-ending injuries. Because baseball is fairly unusual among team sports in how very specialized several of its positions are, my primary concern is with the unique challenges of the pitcher and the risks and injuries specific to his position.

Today, according to Little League rules, a young pitcher who throws fifty-one to sixty-five pitches must wait three days before he can pitch again. The goal is to help prevent overuse injuries that can permanently damage the growing joints, muscles, bones, and ligaments of adolescent athletes; in other words, it's a serious matter. But I have to admit that the story behind the regulation is hardly as grim.

When I entered into talks with the Little League organization in 2009 regarding pitching schedules, I pushed for players to have a minimum of four days off between taking the mound. League administrators and coaches resisted so drastic a measure, knowing that talented pitchers are a valuable commodity for any team. They countered with a standard three-day rest period between games, which they felt was still a major concession on their part. I quickly agreed to the proposal and it was put in the rulebook, but I had to laugh afterward because each party felt that it had won a major victory.

What Little League didn't know was that I didn't have any hard science to back up my push for four days off; I just knew that it was significantly better than no rest at all. So when the League offered up three days as a compromise, I was delighted to agree. It was, undoubtedly, a great starting point!

One of the main focuses of the STOP campaign is to address these needs in youth baseball. Each year in the United States, an estimated sixteen million boys play some form of organized baseball. Five million of them play in an organized youth baseball league outside of school, many of which have no mandated rules and regulations for preventing injuries. The rise of reported injuries for this age group has grown significantly and has generated concern and alarm among pediatric and sports medicine professionals. Of the sixteen million youth baseball participants, it is estimated that 7 to 20 percent between the ages of nine and fifteen will suffer an injury requiring medical attention, with the total estimated medical costs for these injuries at close to $1.8 billion. The overwhelming number of injuries stems from the fact that many baseball players play their one sport year-round on multiple teams. In addition, these children are at risk for sports-related overuse injuries as a result of improper technique, poorly fitting protective equipment, training errors, muscle weakness, and imbalance.

There are many risk factors for youth baseball injuries, but the most compelling research points to the fact that overuse injuries arising from the repetitive microtrauma of small injuries can lead to major injuries.

The incidence of throwing injuries correlates directly with pitching frequency and is higher for pitchers with improper technique. Young athletes are at an increased risk for growth plate injuries, overuse injuries, and heat illness, all of which can be prevented. Young athletes' skeletal maturity, size, coordination, and flexibility put them at increased risk for unique acute and chronic injuries to their bony growth plates that can sometimes result in permanent deformities and dysfunction. Often these injuries do not show up as significant conditions at a young age but become progressively more compounded and recognizable in late adolescence and adulthood. These injuries occur so early in a young athlete's career that they can decrease the opportunities for playing at a higher level of competition later on.

Scientific literature from our American Sports Medicine Institute (ASMI) found four main risk factors for youth baseball injuries: the number of pitches thrown, pitching mechanics, pitch type, and the physical condition of the player.

Excessive Pitch Counts

The number of pitches thrown has the strongest correlation to youth pitching injuries. Many independent and travel teams have no rules restricting pitch counts, or setting guidelines for limits, days of rest, or the cumulative amount of pitching a young pitcher can do. With some leagues and school teams increasing demand on youth athletes to pitch more, there is less time for repairing soft tissues in the elbow and shoulder. Adolescent pitchers who pitched competitively more than eight months out of the year were five times more likely to sustain an elbow or shoulder injury. Individuals who averaged more than eighty-five pitches per outing were four times more likely to develop an injury. And according to a recent report published by ASMI in the *American Journal of Sports Medicine,* those who pitched regularly despite experiencing arm fatigue were *thirty-five* times more likely to injure themselves.

A 2001 study of youth baseball pitchers ages nine to fourteen showed that the odds of elbow pain increased 35 percent when a youngster

- threw seventy-five to ninety-nine pitches per game; or
- exceeded six hundred pitches in a single season; or
- threw certain types of pitches that are known to be taxing on young arms.

The study also revealed that for every ten pitches thrown over a total of seventy-five, the odds of shoulder pain increased dramatically. In fact, the pitchers who threw between seventy-five and ninety-nine pitches per game faced a 52 percent increased risk of shoulder pain.

Youth Baseball Elbow and Youth Baseball Shoulder

The two most common injuries in youth baseball are youth baseball elbow and youth baseball shoulder. Youth baseball elbow (medial epicondyle apophysitis) causes elbow pain while throwing and is exacerbated by throwing harder or farther for longer periods of time. Youth baseball shoulder (proximal humeral epiphysitis), or injury to the growth plate (see chapter 22 for more about growth plate injuries), produces gradual-onset shoulder pain that may increase as the velocity and duration of pitching increases. While overuse is the most compounding risk factor for baseball injuries, many problems begin with improper throwing mechanics. A follow-up study in 2002 found that breaking pitches along with high pitch counts significantly increased the risk of elbow and shoulder pain among youth baseball pitchers ages nine to fourteen. In yet another study of nine- to fourteen-year-old baseball players by ASMI, curveballs were associated with a 52 percent increased risk in shoulder pain, while sliders had an 86 percent increased risk in elbow pain. However, no matter how poor a pitcher's mechanics are or how varied the types of pitches may be, injury is usually the result of repeated "insult" to the elbow and shoulder joint in almost every single throw to the plate.

Although the number of participants in youth baseball has increased, the physical fitness level of the average American youth has declined. The retired MLB great and famously unfit John Kruk once quipped, "I'm a baseball player, not an athlete." Humorous as the statement is, it's not exactly true. Though baseball may require a different kind of fitness than other sports that are more endurance based, physical fitness is still an important part of baseball. Children who are fit excel in baseball and tend to play it with higher frequency. What is true, however, is that unfit children are playing more baseball as well. Proper conditioning, preseason screening, and physicals that check for adequate fitness levels will help decrease injuries caused by poor physical fitness.

Preventing Acute Impact Injuries

Unfortunately, injuries to the elbow and shoulder are not the only injuries that youth baseball players face. In fact, half of all youth baseball league acute injuries are caused by impact with a ball, with 68 percent of injuries occurring on defense.

According to the Consumer Product Safety Commission, eighty-eight baseball-related deaths occurred between 1973 and 1995. Forty-three percent were from direct ball-to-chest impact; 24 percent from direct ball-to-head impact; 15 percent from being struck by a bat; 10 percent from direct ball contact with the neck, ear, or throat; and 8 percent were unknown. Most of these injuries could have been prevented with the use of proper baseball equipment. Also important to note is that baseball is the leading cause of sports-related eye injuries in children ages five to fourteen, with one-third of injuries resulting from being struck by a pitched ball. The US Centers for Disease Control and Prevention (CDC) estimates that half of all sports injuries in children are preventable with proper education and the use of protective equipment. For instance, wearing a metal or plastic face guard can reduce the risk of facial injury by up to 35 percent. In spite of these findings, the use of face guards is not widespread. Therefore, I strongly recommend a universal mandate of face guard usage, as well as the use of safety or reduced-impact balls. The Consumer Product Safety Commission estimates that 32 percent of all injuries, including head injuries and skull fractures, could be prevented by the use of these balls. Self-protective measures can also prevent tragedies from happening, such as a batter's knowing to turn away from an oncoming ball; not kneeling in the on-deck circle, where you can easily be struck by a foul ball or a wild pitch; and being instructed in proper sliding techniques.

With help from the STOP Sports Injury Campaign, our goal is that seminars focused on injury prevention will protect young athletes and improve their opportunity for success at a higher performance level.

Managing Baseball-Related Injuries

The fact of the matter is, if a young athlete is throwing too hard, too much, too early, and without rest, a serious elbow or shoulder injury may be on the horizon. If the athlete complains of elbow or shoulder pain the day after throwing, or joint movement is painful or restricted compared with the opposite side, he should try "active rest"—that is, remaining active while ceasing activity for the affected body part—and, if necessary, see a physician familiar with youth sports injuries.

Applying ice to the hurt area reduces soreness and inflammation. Ibuprofen, a nonsteroidal anti-inflammatory drug, or NSAID, can help relieve any pain. If symptoms persist, it is critical that a physician be contacted, especially if there is a lack of full-joint motion. An examination and X-rays should be conducted. An MRI scan may also be helpful. Remember, though, that a sophisticated imaging test such as an MRI or a CT scan (short for computerized tomography) does not take the place of a physician's keeping comprehensive records of a patient's history, along with a thorough physical exam and routine X-rays.

Usually a simple rest-cure approach will not be enough, because even though it allows symptoms to subside, the spell of inactivity also leads to a loss of muscle bulk, tone, flexibility, and endurance. Once the pain is gone and full motion returns, a throwing rehabilitation program can start. Under more severe circumstances, surgery may be necessary to correct a problem. Overuse and stress-related problems can affect growing parts of the bone, not just the soft tissue (muscles, tendons, and ligaments). If the condition is not treated, it could cause deformity of the limb and permanent disability. The athlete should return to play only when clearance is granted by a health care professional.

Preventing Overuse Injuries

Overuse injuries—especially those related to the ulnar collateral ligament (UCL) of the elbow and the rotator cuff and labrum of the shoulder—are preventable. By practicing smart, a player can prolong his career exponentially. In pitching, as in most things, quality is vastly more important than quantity. Throwing fewer pitches with greater concentration and body awareness does far more for developing talent than simply hurling a ball for hours. As my good friend and mentor to many young baseball players Hall of Famer Hank Aaron often says, "Learn to pitch by throwing strikes and placing the ball. Don't worry about velocity and breaking balls at a young age." If the great Hank Aaron stands by that philosophy, you know it is sound advice!

In order to make the most of any practice, it is important to follow some valuable guidelines. Start with a proper warm-up that gets the heart pumping and stretches muscles. Also, pitching should always start out with easy throws, building gradually to full-strength hurling. If the athlete experiences any elbow or shoulder pain that does not go away after stretching and a few easy practice throws, he should stop immediately. If the pain persists longer than a few days, consult a doctor. Be sure that there is open communication between the player and the coach regarding how an arm feels. Coaches should be alert to any visible signs of fatigue or pain, such as the player rubbing or massaging the arm between throws or wincing during the windup or release. The athlete himself needs to be responsible for his well-being, too, however, as he is the only one who can truly assess the way his arm feels. If there is pain, he must feel that he can tell his coach and remove himself from the game without fearing he will be penalized in the future.

It is important that pitchers focus on throwing with proper technique, maintain control over their body, and aim for accuracy over speed; nothing burns out an arm more quickly than sloppy mechanics resulting from trying to clock a higher mph. I recommend that radar guns should never be used in youth sports; it's simply not necessary or appropriate for twelve-year-olds to be concerned with precisely how fast each pitch is crossing the plate. The use of such guns only adds pressure and the potential for overuse, as a child's natural tendency is to think, "Just one more throw; maybe I can break my record this time!" Instead, coaches and parents should be concerned with age-appropriate skills, encouraging young pitchers under the age of thirteen to master the fastball and changeup before attempting any breaking pitches. Until the fundamental groundwork is laid for executing proper form with the simple pitches, nothing requiring more specialized wrist motions or fancy snaps should even be considered.

Pitchers should also adhere to age-appropriate pitch-count and mandatory-rest guidelines as established by their league. As of 2010, the Little League baseball regular season and tournament pitching rules have established clear guidelines for acceptable pitch counts and time off between games. Remember that more sophisticated pitches such as curveballs, sliders, and so on require more sophisticated neuromuscular control—and that comes only with age.

For pitchers age fourteen and under, rest requirements are as follows:

- If a player throws sixty-six or more pitches in a day: four calendar days of rest.
- If a player throws fifty-one to sixty-five pitches in a day: three calendar days of rest.
- If a player throws thirty-six to fifty pitches in a day: two calendar days of rest.
- If a player throws twenty-one to thirty-five pitches in a day: one calendar day of rest.
- If a player throws one to twenty pitches in a day: no rest required.

For league players between fifteen and eighteen years of age, the pitch counts and rest periods are slightly different:

- If a player throws seventy-six or more pitches in a day: four calendar days of rest.
- If a player throws sixty-one to seventy-five pitches in a day: three calendar days of rest.
- If a player throws forty-six to sixty pitches in a day: two calendar days of rest.
- If a player throws thirty-one to forty-five pitches in a day: one calendar day of rest.
- If a player pitches one to thirty pitches in a day: no rest required.

Clearly, pitching on consecutive days for the same team is out of the question. However, some athletes try to get around this by playing in multiple leagues during the same season. They often reason that more playing time means more practice, but just the opposite is true. Any pitcher playing for more than one competitive league in the same season runs the risk of overuse injuries, besides simply becoming burnt out on the sport.

It is also advisable that parents and coaches encourage pitchers between ages nine and fourteen to throw the fastball and changeup exclusively and not throw the curveball or slider. A good rule of thumb is that "you should not throw a breaking ball—for example, a curveball—until you shave." That means that the young baseball player has progressed well into puberty and his bones, growth plates, and articular cartilage surfaces have all matured.

Around the Horn

I recommend strongly that all youth baseball players, not just pitchers, consider playing other positions. Not only does this help keep them involved in the game, but they'll also learn the strategy of each position and develop different skill sets on the diamond. More important, it keeps them from overworking any one set of muscles or joints to the point of injury. The challenges for pitchers are clear, but consider some of the other positions. The catcher ranks right below the pitcher in risking injury. For example, he can develop knee, feet, or hip problems from the sustained crouching position if he allows his knees to roll inward or if he shifts the bulk of his weight to one side or another for a prolonged period. Encouraging him to play the occasional game in the outfield or at shortstop can hone his reflexes as well as allow his legs to stretch and move in a more natural manner.

Catchers' health concerns are not often highlighted but must be taken into consideration. He's usually the only player who throws more in the game than the pitcher. While he doesn't need to focus on the velocity of every throw as much, he still has to hurl the ball either back to the mound or to a base after every pitch. It's kind of like the old expression about the famous film dance partners Fred Astaire and Ginger Rogers: "Everything Fred Astaire did, Ginger Rogers did backward and in heels." Everything a pitcher does, a catcher has to do, but while crouching and wearing what is, essentially, a suit of armor. If a catcher complains of shoulder or elbow pain, it should be taken seriously and treated in the same manner as a pitching injury caused by overuse. Undoubtedly, one of the craziest cases I have ever seen was a fifteen-year-old catcher who tore his UCL at a baseball tryout. This catcher was among a number of other young men playing the same position who were asked to throw one hundred baseballs to second base as hard and as fast as they could in two hundred seconds. Not every participant was able to make the maximum number of throws in two hundred seconds. Around the fiftieth throw, the teen's elbow ligament actually split in half.

The following additional recommendations are supported by research from the Medical Advisory Committee of USA Baseball, the national governing body for amateur baseball, and in partnership with the American Sports Medicine Institute:

Awareness
- Be aware of common overuse injuries associated with baseball pitchers.
- Educate parents that pain plus tenderness, especially in a joint, are often signs of overuse and should not be ignored.

- Educate parents about Little League baseball's new pitching rules and regulations.
- Encourage parents to monitor pitch counts and required rest periods based on their child's age.
- Watch for and respond to signs of fatigue.
- If a youth pitcher complains of fatigue or looks fatigued, let him or her rest from pitching and other throwing.
- Youth pitchers should learn good throwing mechanics as soon as possible. The first steps should be to learn, in order: (1) basic throwing, (2) fastball pitching, and (3) changeup pitching.
- Preseason physicals are important for detecting preexisting health risks.
- Adequate hydration is essential.
- Prevention is the key!

Warming Up
- Make sure that parents and coaches give their children enough time to warm up properly and stretch before and after play. (Cold muscles are more prone to injury.)

Rules and Regulations
- Follow limits for pitch counts and days of rest. (Pitch counts should be monitored and regulated.)
- Avoid using radar guns.
- Youth sports leagues should provide and require first aid training for coaches. (This training could be performed by sports medicine professionals and include recognition and immediate response to head, neck, and spine injuries, as well as heat-related illnesses.)
- Youth sports leagues should have clear, enforceable return-to-play guidelines for concussions, neck and back injuries, fractures, and dislocations.
- Proper equipment (including face guards on batting helmets) and field surface conditions should be required.

- Pitchers should not throw breaking pitches (curveballs, sliders) in competition until their bones have matured (around thirteen years old).
- Pitchers should be discouraged from participating in tryout showcases.
- Medical coverage should be present at all sporting events.
- Proper officiating can keep all players using safe-play techniques.

Checking Out the Coach
- Parents should ask the team's coach if he utilizes drills to minimize the risk of injury and if he follows Little League baseball pitching rules.
- Coaches should adhere to all injury-prevention recommendations and have proper training.

Cross-Training
- Children should be encouraged to play a different sport each season that utilizes different muscle groups. For example, pitchers should avoid swimming, tennis, and playing quarterback in football, as these utilize the same muscle groups. They would be much better served by allowing their shoulders and elbows a chance to recover.
- Children should avoid participating on more than one sports team at a time.
- A pitcher should not also play catcher for his or her team. The two positions are equally taxing on young throwing arms.
- Pitchers should be discouraged from returning to the mound after already having been removed as the pitcher to avoid overworking the pitching arm.
- Inspire youth pitchers to have fun playing baseball and other sports.
- Participation in and enjoyment of various physical activities will increase the youth's athleticism and interest in sports.

Taking Breaks
- Children who focus solely on baseball need to take time to recover each year.
- Players should avoid pitching more than eight months out of the year because of increased risk of injuries requiring surgery.
- Mandate a three-consecutive-months-rest period each year for throwing athletes.

Don't Ignore Arm or Elbow Pain!
- Children should never pitch if they feel arm pain or fatigue. Pitchers who pitch despite arm fatigue are three to six times more vulnerable to injury.
- If a pitcher complains of pain in his or her elbow, get an evaluation from a sports medicine physician.

Parents should remember that there are different kinds of fatigue that may affect their child: year-round fatigue (never taking any time off), seasonal fatigue (overworking the arm over a period of several weeks or months), and event fatigue (overly intensive work over a period of a few hours or days).

It's the great American pastime, and for good reason: Athletes learn the merits of playing as part of a team but also have a chance to display their individual talents. Baseball has always been considered a safe sport, and it is the responsibility of all involved adults to keep it that way.

My hope for baseball, as with all youth sports, is that regulations and precautions do not hamper the game with too many rules but allow young athletes to participate in the sport for as long as possible. I want to see kids who are excited to grab a mitt and take the field, not ones who are wincing in pain at the thought of playing another inning. I want to see a new generation of baseball players who grow up loving the game and keeping their bodies healthy not only into young adulthood but well beyond.

For all of us involved in the medical aspects of sports, it is our obligation to promote health and wellness as well as to educate and apply prevention strategies when necessary. By educating coaches, parents, and youth baseball players, the common incidences of preventable injuries will decrease. It is our hope that all community baseball leagues will follow in Little League's footsteps and implement the recommended safety guidelines.

Chapter 6
Basketball

It's hard to beat the excitement of a high school gym on a doubleheader Friday night. Sometimes it's the junior varsity at six o'clock and the varsity at eight; sometimes it's the women's varsity followed by the men's varsity. The smell of the polished gym floor and of popcorn popping at the concession stand, the sound of the buzzer and stomping feet on the bleachers during an opponent's free throw—those are part of the magic of basketball that takes us all back to memories of high school or church leagues or community teams or maybe just shooting hoops in the driveway or at the local rec center. It doesn't require any special gear or even much equipment to play. In some communities, high school basketball is the center of local social activity, and in some towns, girls' basketball even outdraws its male counterpart! Every March, when the NCAA tournament brackets come out, we hear about "Cinderella teams" from smaller schools that have a shot at the national spotlight. There is a reason that basketball is one of the best-loved sports in America. Well over a half million boys hit the court each year, and girls are closing the gap, nearing 460,000 participants nationwide.

Unfortunately, girls' basketball clocks in even higher than boys' when it comes to injuries, and women's basketball is currently a hot topic in sports medicine. This is great news for young female basketball players because it means that more attention is being given to the prevention and treatment of their injuries. I have to admit, though, that despite the fact that approximately 1.6 million basketball injuries are reported each year, I'm still shocked that the high-energy, fast-moving, contact/collision nature of this sport doesn't produce more complex injuries than it does. That tells me that parents and coaches are doing something right; however, there is still much that can be done to protect these children.

The most commonly hurt area for basketball players is the lower leg, and ankle sprains are especially common. While most sprains can be effectively treated by the RICE approach (rest, ice, compression, and elevation), a doctor should be consulted if there is swelling or bruising over the bone, as this might indicate a more serious injury. Wrist sprains can also occur if a falling player tries to break his fall with his hand. Since a wrist unable to execute a full range of motion is clearly a disadvantage when trying to shoot the ball, this can be a very frustrating injury for any player to endure. Coaches and players must remember, though, that just because a joint is sprained rather than broken, the injury should *not* be shrugged off. Ankle sprains are serious injuries, even if they are not as severe as fractures. No athlete should ever be forced to play with a sprained ankle—it can exacerbate the existing injury and cause secondary injuries, as athletes compensate for the pain. The athlete should expect to spend a minimum of a week out of the game for a sprain, although two or three weeks are reasonable for more severe sprains.

Stress fractures in the foot and lower leg also result from overuse, often following the first few weeks of the season, when the player pushes to reach last season's peak training marks too quickly. If the child begins to feel pain in the bone during or after practice, he or she should stop activity and rest the leg or foot until it has fully healed, because continuing to play heightens the risk of reinjuring the bone or causing a stress fracture. The same is true of fatiguing the wrist joint if the child is committed to perfecting free throws by practicing for hours on end. Athletes must remember that conditioning occurs gradually and that a steady buildup in activity level will yield much better results than trying to immediately jump back into a full-blown workout routine after time off.

Basketball, like so many other sports, is a cutting game, which means that the knee is at an elevated risk for injury. ACL tears are fairly common in basketball, especially among girls, and can result from either a sharp shift in the body's momentum while dribbling the ball or playing defense, or landing wrong following a jump shot. This is an extremely painful injury that requires surgical repair; players will usually report feeling a *pop* or *snap* in their knee as the ligament rips from the impact. The athlete will usually not be able to walk following such an injury and will need assistance leaving the court. If she cannot put any weight on the joint upon standing, under no circumstances should she attempt to get around on her own. Unfortunately, the postsurgical recovery time for an ACL tear generally is around six to twelve months. The good news is that most are not career ending, and the athlete should be able to play again the following year. Of course, that is hardly good news to a teenager who wants to get back out with his or her team right away. The only option is to funnel that energy toward rehabilitation therapy.

The other problem with a basketball-induced ACL injury is that the constant joint pounding and twisting from playing on the hardwood floor often produces associated trauma in other areas of the knee, such as cartilage injuries or meniscus tears. Another serious and quite painful injury caused by cutting is patellar (kneecap) dislocation. This injury can be as devastating as an ACL injury and can cause permanent damage to the patella and even bone and joint growth. It often requires surgical correction. Bruising of the knee can occur when the outside of the joint is struck or endures hard impact with the floor or ball and can cause temporary dysfunction. Rest and ice can help to bring the swelling and pain under control, while a knee brace will help to stabilize the joint while the athlete recovers. Once the pain has subsided and the full range of motion has returned, the player can ease back into practice or games.

Simple strengthening and flexibility exercises (see chapter 32) can help the body protect the joint by allowing it a greater range of motion and also forming a kind of natural, protective brace around vulnerable joints and their components. For this reason, a thorough and targeted warm-up that works each major muscle group is extremely important.

Since basketball is primarily a winter sport, players will sometimes hit the court from cold temperatures outside, which leaves them more vulnerable to pulls and tears. Some teams allow players to conduct their warm-up routines independently before starting drills as a team. Talk with your child's coach about the best exercises for your youngster to prepare the joints and muscles for practice or play. Have him arrive at practice a few minutes early for a little extra time to get the blood flowing. Even five additional minutes of good, joint-specific stretching can make the difference between a good game and an injury.

Not all injuries will knock a player out of action for the duration of the game. When the ball strikes the end of the fingers, causing a joint to swell, the finger may be iced and then buddy wrapped with an adjacent finger—a kind of natural splint that the body provides—and the player can return to the court as soon as he or she feels ready. The player should never be forced to return, however, if the pain is too intense; nor should the injury be ignored if there is any visible bruising or the finger is bent at an unnatural angle. These are signs of a much more serious injury, such as a fracture, and professional medical attention should be sought, as an X-ray may be necessary for a more complete diagnosis.

Athletes should also be cautious about any lacerations they might encounter while playing. Because basketball is played in such close contact with so little protective equipment, the chance of getting cut by an opponent's fingernail or metal orthodontic braces is quite high. Most cuts are very minor and can be cleaned and dressed with a simple adhesive bandage. If a deeper cut occurs, however, it may be necessary to close it with butterfly tape. The athletic trainer should have this in the team's first aid kit, and the player can return to the game as soon as the bleeding has stopped and he feels comfortable getting back on the court. Should any blood spill on the floor of the court, play should be suspended briefly while it is cleaned and the area disinfected. Rarely, a cut may be serious enough to require stitches, but most contact in basketball should be incidental enough that such a deep laceration is unlikely.

I recommend the following guidelines for both boys' and girls' basketball teams in order to ensure the best and safest possible playing experience for everyone involved:

1. As with any major youth sport, athletes should undergo a pre-season physical examination by a pediatrician or family practice doctor.

2. Basketball players should hydrate adequately. They should also pay attention to weather advisories in order to avoid heat-related illness.

3. Those participating in basketball should maintain proper fitness and should have a gradual preseason workup to get in shape before they begin active basketball competition.

4. Athletes should avoid overtraining in order to stave off overuse injuries such as stress fractures.

5. Players should listen to their bodies and decrease training time and/or intensity if pain develops. This will reduce the risk of injury and help avoid burnout. I know it's hard for players to voluntarily bench themselves, but it will serve both the player and the team better in the long run if they are honest about any pain they are feeling.

6. The use of an athletic trainer at all levels of youth basketball is encouraged. Athletic trainers are especially needed at all youth basketball practices. If there are any questions related to a specific injury to a youth basketball player, an evaluation by a certified athletic trainer should be conducted, followed by a referral to a sports medicine physician when appropriate.

Basketball has been a favorite ever since James Naismith first nailed a peach basket to the wall of a Springfield, Massachusetts, YMCA in 1891. Popular among many families, as boys and girls can practice together at home with just a hoop in the driveway, it is a great sport that can help athletes develop hand-eye coordination and cardiovascular health, as well as team building and self-esteem. If parents and grandparents take the time to educate themselves about the potential risks, and encourage their budding athletes to take the best steps to protect themselves and stay healthy, basketball can provide a lifetime of fitness, fun, and recreation.

Chapter 7
Cheerleading

I've seen cheerleaders proudly wearing shirts emblazed with the slogan "If cheerleading was any easier, they would call it football." That's no exaggeration! Cheerleading has evolved far beyond what its name has implied in years past: a group of peppy men and women leading cheers from the sidelines to support the team and fire up the crowd. While this is still true in some leagues, in many places the focus has shifted from school spirit to flashy displays of dance, gymnastics, and acrobatics. It is certainly exciting to watch and a great opportunity for young people to be active. However, the recent trend toward throws and stunts has greatly increased the injury factor. Because of this, I do not believe it is an exaggeration to say that cheerleading is completely out of control.

Unfortunately, many parents don't understand the risks associated with cheerleading because it was a much tamer sport in generations past. In fact, many people used to scoff (and still do) at the notion that cheerleading could be considered a sport at all. I would beg to differ. Cheerleading requires all kinds of highly athletic movements, with a mix of dance and gymnastic skills as well as complex stunt and pyramid maneuvers. Furthermore, it now has an almost inevitable competitive component, as teams perform in contests that rate their routines on synchronization, spirit, form, and difficulty. As the father of a cheerleader, I can testify to the long hours and intense practices these young people undergo, which makes them as entitled to the designation of "athlete" as anyone.

In 2002, an estimated three and a half million people in the United States participated in cheerleading, and the number has grown steadily since then. Cheerleaders now begin performing at an earlier age. No longer is it confined to high school and college teams. While boys usually join the sport a bit older and stop after college, girls are now participating on teams at ages as young as four, and many seek to continue into adulthood as cheerleaders for professional athletic teams.

With the complexity and competitive nature that cheerleading has developed, both the injury rates and the potential for severe injury have increased. Statistics show that cheerleading accounts for more than sixteen thousand emergency room visits annually in the United States, and *more than half* the catastrophic injuries in female athletes. In 1982 the National Center for Catastrophic Sport Injury Research (NCCSIR) initiated an annual catastrophic injury report that compiles statistics on fatalities, disabilities, and serious injuries from high school and collegiate sports in the United States. Initially, cheerleading was not even included until two collegiate cheerleaders suffered serious head injuries during the first year of data collection. From 1982 through 2008, collegiate cheerleading was associated with thirty-one catastrophic injuries and high school cheerleading with seventy-three. During this time, cheerleading accounted for 70.5 percent of college women's catastrophic sports injuries and 65.2 percent of all high school female catastrophic sports injuries.

As I mentioned on page 4, the NCAA reports that the total health insurance costs associated with collegiate cheerleading make up fully 25 percent of the overall medical costs. That's higher than the total for nearly ninety other sports combined. Although college football accounts for 57 percent of the total medical costs, it also has ten times the participation of cheerleading. Cheerleaders are prone to many injuries typical of youth sports, such as sprains and strains; however, it is unique in just how large a percentage of its injuries are serious—especially to the head and neck. Skull fractures, concussions, cervical spine injuries resulting in quadriplegia, lower spine injuries resulting in paraplegia, and even death can occur if stunts are not properly executed or supervised. While the flyers (the person at the top of the stunt or in the air for the throw) are usually the focus of concern, the bases (the people who do the lifting or throwing) are at risk as well. If the flyer lands incorrectly, they risk impacting the base's shoulder or neck. Certified mats should be made mandatory; parents should not be afraid to ask about the mats used in their child's practices. There should also be an automated external defibrillator (AED) at the practice facility that is checked regularly to be in working order and holding a charge.

Fatigue is a major factor, as routines are performed over and over to achieve perfection; however, the repetition can become counterproductive if it goes on too long. Cheerleaders should not attempt a complex stunt if they are tired, injured, or ill, as even the slightest instability can make it an unsafe maneuver. Because every member of the team is required for stunts and choreography formations, many coaches are reluctant to remove a cheerleader nursing a sprain, choosing instead to have him or her brace the injury and continue competing. Under no circumstances should an athlete with a healing injury have any participation in stunts; if he or she is part of a stunt, the routine must be adapted to something not requiring the involvement of the injured person but still involving the required number of participants for safe execution.

If a fall should occur that results in a spinal injury, the athlete *should not be lifted or moved in any way* except by medical professionals. Signs and symptoms that there may be a spinal injury are loss of consciousness; numbness, tingling, or radiating pain in the extremities; pain directly over the spine; confusion or inability to answer simple questions; blood and/ or spinal fluid leaking from the ears or nose; difficulty breathing; inability to move the extremities; and/or memory loss. Improper movement can result in permanent paralysis or death. All cheerleading competitions should have an emergency response team on site; ideally, the same is true for practices, but this is not likely. The program should have a risk management plan and strategies to promote all aspects of safety. Parents should familiarize themselves with this plan as well. At least one person should be present at all times who is certified in advanced life-saving techniques, with special emphasis on spinal injury. If it is established that rescue breathing is necessary, the person with the most medical training should deliver the breaths in such a way that requires a minimal amount of movement to the head and neck. It goes without saying that the routine or practice ends immediately.

Even if a fall does not result in catastrophic harm, there is still the chance that a serious injury could have occurred. When a cheerleader shows signs of head trauma, such as a loss of consciousness, visual disturbances, headaches, an inability to walk correctly, nausea or vomiting, obvious disorientation, and/or memory loss, he or she should receive immediate medical attention and should not be allowed to practice or cheer without written permission from a physician. It is important to remember that an athlete can have a concussion or other serious brain injury without losing consciousness.

Age guidelines have been put into place by several of the major national cheerleading organizations that limit pyramids and other stunts in different age groups to two body lengths for the high school level and two and a half body lengths for the collegiate level, with the base cheerleader remaining in direct contact with the performing surface. Also, base supporters must remain stationary and the suspended person or persons may not be inverted or rotated on dismount.

Stunt-specific recommendations also encompass the thrower-to-flyer ratio and the number of spotters for each person lifted above shoulder level. For example, basket toss stunts—in which a cheerleader is thrown into the air, sometimes as high as twenty feet—are allowed to have no more than four throwers. The person being tossed is not allowed to drop her head below a horizontal plane with her torso, and one of the throwers must remain under the flyer at all times during the toss. Unfortunately, while these rules are a great starting point for protecting the athletes, they are largely abandoned at the higher levels of competition, as squads push boundaries more and more for the "wow factor" in their routines.

The National Federation of State High School Associations (NFHS) and the NCAA should formally make cheerleading a sport, which would place it under the same restrictions and safety rules as all other high school and collegiate sports; unfortunately, this effort has recently hit some roadblocks, which I will discuss below. All high school cheerleading coaches should be familiar with the *NFHS Spirit Rules Book,* updated annually, and should always have it available for reference before attempting any stunt. Collegiate coaches should have a copy of the *AACCA Cheerleading Safety Manual,* from the American Association of Cheerleading Coaches and Administrators, and be familiar with its contents. These books are also important resources for independent competitive cheerleading squads and should be read thoroughly by those coaches.

The numerous competitive cheerleading squads that are staples in many cities and small towns have become more and more athletically demanding and potentially more dangerous on a yearly basis. This is due to the intense competition at all levels, and the belief that the earlier a child gets started, the better his or her chances are for a future in the sport. Obviously, these new dynamics bring about an increased risk of injury; thus, the need for rules and regulations relative to pyramiding and stunting and the role of the flyer in pyramid stunting.

The NCCSIR recommends the following safety measures:

- Cheerleaders should have a medical examination, including a complete medical history, before they are allowed to participate.
- Cheerleaders should be trained by qualified coaches with cheerleading certification and training in gymnastics and partner stunting. He or he should also be trained in the proper methods for spotting and other safety factors.
- Cheerleaders should be exposed to proper conditioning programs and trained in proper spotting techniques.
- Cheerleaders should receive proper training before attempting gymnastics and partner stunts, and should not attempt stunts they are not capable of completing. A qualified system demonstrating mastery of stunts is recommended.
- Coaches should supervise all practice sessions in a safe facility.
- Many routines involving trampolines and flips or falls off pyramids should be prohibited.

- Pyramids should not be higher than two people, and pyramids in general should not be performed without mats and proper spotting.
- If it is not possible to have a physician or certified athletic trainer at games and practice sessions, emergency procedures should be provided by the school or cheer organization. The emergency plan should be displayed prominently and be available in writing to everyone involved in the program, including the athletes.

I support these recommendations wholeheartedly. The problem is that they are just that: recommendations, not hard-and-fast rules that all squads must follow. Cheerleading can certainly be made safer, and understanding the risk factors will undoubtedly make it a more productive sport for the participants. Proper supervision and proper spotters, along with certified mats and good coaching, are the cornerstones for combating injury. Mats should, of course, be used during all practice sessions and competitions (except when cheering on a rubberized track), but a mat can provide only so much protection when a person falls from a height of ten feet or more. Likewise, adult spotters should always be employed until a stunt or tumbling pass can be performed with confidence and without error a minimum of ten consecutive times. Squads of elementary school–aged cheerleaders should have an adult spotter familiar with the routine—not just another cheerleader—present for all stunts, even during competition.

The importance of a qualified and certified coach is critical. She should be well versed in proper techniques for executing stunts and tumbling and have a thorough knowledge of first aid. She should take into account weather factors when cheering outdoors and cancel stunt routines when conditions are wet. Coaches should also have a realistic grasp on age-appropriate routines in terms of difficulty and the amount of time required in practice; parents may also consider watching other teams from the same gym to make sure that the choreography is age appropriate. Parents should not be shy about asking to see the coaches' certifications at their local cheer gym. If you do not feel comfortable with the credentials of those supervising your child, look for a different team.

Obviously, cheerleading is a great sport, and by promoting safety, it will continue to grow in popularity. Thanks to the coordinated efforts of parents, coaches, participants, and the sports medicine community, injury rates among cheerleaders have dropped dramatically. (The lower numbers, however, cover only high school teams and do not account for all-star, gym-based teams.) There is further good news to report: Recently, the number of catastrophic injuries reported to the NCCSI in cheerleading has been declining steadily, with only three such injuries reported in 2011. This is not to say that any number of horrible injuries is ever acceptable; however, the world of cheerleading has recognized the injury risk associated with the sport and is actively trying to prevent injuries through education, training, and regulation.

In the interest of increasing the safety of cheerleading as a sport, USA Cheer brought the American Association of Cheerleading Coaches and Administrators under its umbrella. AACCA has recently created a certification process by which coaches can learn the most current safety standards in this sport. All of the things that I have talked about in the first part of this chapter are now standard and required prevention mandates. The effort that AACCA has made in certifying coaches is also a big step forward. This certification requires knowledge of the mechanics of cheers and stunts, as well as proper warm-up techniques, dietary needs, rest periods, talent assessment, gym organizations, an emergency management plan, insurance, transportation, and many other topics. The purpose of bringing the two groups together was to increase quality standards among coaches and gymnasiums, as well as to create a standard certification for coaches from the standpoints of both safety and quality.

Currently, AACCA's certification is required by many states for its high school cheerleading coaches, and it is considered the industry standard for safety certification in the sport. This has become such a hot topic that, along with the American Sports Medicine Institute in Birmingham, USA Cheer and AACCA are now hosting a national Cheerleading Safety

Symposium designed to gather some of the leaders in sports medicine along with the leading coaches, athletes, and gym owners to share and exchange information related to current techniques, injury patterns, and, most important, injury prevention. The symposium has been headed by one of my orthopedic sports medicine colleagues, Dr. Jeff Dugas, who is the medical director of USA Cheer.

One of the major issues at hand is the lack of standardization rules among competitive organizations. Some allow athletes to perform stunts and skills that others prohibit. As athletes and coaches search for ways to distinguish themselves to impress high-level coaches, they may choose to participate in competition where rules banning certain maneuvers are not in effect. This is similar to a youth baseball league that lacks pitch limits: Athletes will eventually get hurt. It is a shame for any organization to use the lack of safety rules and regulations as a promotional tool to lure parents and young athletes to its program.

In 2010, a federal judge in Connecticut found that sideline collegiate cheerleading was not a sport, based on the premise that the primary role of cheerleaders is not a competitive one. Obviously, for all of us involved in the safety of our young athletes, cheerleading is no different from any other sport and therefore should be designated as such. This decision has had an immediate impact on the cheerleading world, and universities can no longer count cheerleaders among scholarship-eligible athletes when dealing with matters that pertain to Title IX. (See chapter 34 for a full discussion about Title IX.)

On the positive side, this has cleared the way for organizations like USA Cheer to create and organize a new sport related to cheerleading called Stunt. The first Stunt competitions took place in 2011, with twenty-two NCAA institutions participating. This number promises to grow as more universities recognize the need for competitive cheerleading programs with rigorous safety regulations. In fact, eight high school athletic associations have Stunt programs and held Stunt competitions in 2012 for the first time. USA Cheer has created a safety council composed of sports medicine experts, along with top-level coaches, administrators, and current members of the Team USA cheerleading team. Through this safety council and the creation of Stunt, USA Cheer is taking a leadership role in cheerleading safety and education by creating a standard set of safety guidelines and rules for competition.

We are all hopeful that cheerleading will be classified as a competitive sport. Such a classification could enhance safety guidelines and create opportunities for NCAA scholarships. In the meantime, USA Cheer is taking measures to decrease injury rates and ensure that cheerleading becomes a safe and healthy event.

Research concerning safety in cheerleading must continue. At the time of publication, the NCAA has an injury data collection system in place for all sports except cheerleading. Cheerleading should also be included as an NCAA athletic event, with the same recognition, safety guidelines, and supervision as all other NCAA events. I urge concerned parents and coaches to write to the organization to ask that such measures be put into place. In the meantime, other organizations are collecting data for study. Catastrophic injuries can be reported to the NCCSIR at mueller@email.unc.edu or to the National Center for Catastrophic Sports Injury Research itself at www.cheerinjuryreport.com. Obviously, cheerleading is a great sport, and by promoting safety, it will continue to grow.

Chapter 8
Cycling

The bicycle was invented in the nineteenth century and grew rapidly into a worldwide phenomenon. Today there are approximately one billion bikes in existence—nearly twice the number of automobiles! While cycling as a primary mode of transportation tends to be found more in other countries, it is growing in popularity in the United States, as more and more commuters are turning to bikes as an environmentally friendly, gasoline-free option. Most Americans, however, still view their bike as a tool for recreation and exercise rather than as a way of life, and that's okay too. Cycling is actually one of the best sports for gradually introducing (or reintroducing) physical activity to someone who has not been active for a while, because it is generally a low-impact sport that provides a great workout while sparing the joints too much wear and tear. It's a regular sight in my rehab clinics: a professional football player recovering from knee surgery pedaling away on a stationary bike to help recondition his muscles and restore the joint's range of motion. But what many people discover after they begin casual cycling for the sake of cardiovascular health or as part of physical therapy is that they really love it and decide to pursue it more aggressively.

The very first thing that any potential cycler should look at is a quality helmet. Even though many states do not have laws requiring them, helmets can cut the rate of head injuries by 85 percent when worn properly. Although a good helmet does not have to be expensive, there are several things that parents should look for when shopping. First, make sure that the helmet fits the head snugly but does not leave red marks on the skin when removed. If a child seems to be in between sizes, buy the larger one, but never buy in anticipation of a growth spurt, as a loose helmet provides far less protection. Also make sure that the child's ears are not obstructed, so that he or she can still discern external sounds easily—such as approaching vehicles and other environmental factors when riding on roads. Make sure, too, that the helmet has a plastic shell. Some lightweight Styrofoam helmets, while providing protection from impact in a fall, can actually cause neck and spine injuries due to their tendency to "grip" the ground upon impact, jarring the bones by absorbing, rather than deflecting, the momentum. Helmets with a slick or smooth outer casing are more likely to slide, even on rough surfaces such as asphalt. The benefit of such a helmet is that in a fall, the energy of the impact is dispersed more fully if the body is able to move with the momentum, which is generally safer for the wearer.

In terms of joint and bone injuries, one of the most common complaints is knee pain as a result of overuse. This is ironic, of course, since cycling is one of the most common forms of rehabilitation exercise for patients recovering from knee injuries caused by other sports. The danger comes from attempting to push the joint too long or at too difficult a level than the muscles and tendons are prepared for. Even healthy riders can run the risk of overdoing it if they push their muscles to the point of fatigue or try to pedal in too high a gear. Patellar tendinitis and patellofemoral syndrome can result when the knee and its surrounding tendons and bones are irritated, producing pain in the kneecap. Iliotibial band friction, which is a thickening of tissue in the thigh and knee, tends to cause pain in the outer knee, but can be treated similarly to kneecap soreness. The first step is to rest and ice the leg to reduce the irritation and any inflammation. When the pain has subsided, consider a flexible brace to help stabilize the joint when returning to the activity. Arch supports in the shoes or wedges on the pedals can also help to alter the positioning of the foot and ankle in such a way that may reduce the amount of stress on the knee. Any bike shop should have several different pedal options. Parents should also limit their children's biking workouts to no longer than an hour a day until they have established a baseline of fitness.

The feet can be a source of pain, tingling, or numbness after especially long or intense rides. Sometimes the solution is as simple as wearing a wider shoe to allow for unrestricted blood flow to the extremity; other times, the pain may be the result of pressure and compression on the nerves of the lower leg, called exertional compartment syndrome. If numbness in the foot becomes a problem, cyclists should first rest their legs and try different shoes. If the condition does not improve, they should consult a physician, as severe cases may warrant surgery to relieve the pressure and prevent nerve or blood vessel damage.

A more delicate location for cycling-related pain is the genital and rectal area. One cause is the proverbial "saddle sores" suffered by cowboys and cyclists alike. These annoying red bumps, almost like acne, will arise on the buttocks as a result of irritated hair follicles. If left untreated, the follicles can develop infections and become painful, pus-filled abscesses. Simple steps to reduce saddle sores include adjusting the bike seat to the optimal height, applying cream or petroleum jelly to the affected area prior to a ride, and wearing cycling gear fitted with padding in the crotch and rear. Chamois padding in pants can also help reduce or even prevent pudendal neuropathy, in which compression of the blood supply to nerves in the genital region generates numbness and pain. This condition can also usually be resolved by adjusting the bicycle seat, either by tilting it to a more comfortable angle or swapping it for a different shape entirely, according to the individual needs of the rider's body.

Neck and back pain are also common complaints after long rides, due largely to the fact that the cyclist must lean forward to grip the handlebars. If the bars are set to low or too high, the rider may have to round or arch the back to compensate. Slowing down briefly to safely turn the head, stretch the neck, and shrug the shoulders can help relax those muscles and keep the blood flowing. Flexibility exercises (see chapter 32) to loosen the hamstrings and the hips can also allow the rider to maintain a comfortable posture without causing undue strain on the lower back.

Sometimes simply switching to a different grip on the handlebar can also prevent the overuse of one set of muscles or joints and can help reduce wrist and forearm pain. Cyclists should never lock their arms but, instead, always ride with their elbows slightly bent, as this will help absorb the shock of any uneven patches or bumps in the road. Carpal tunnel syndrome can occur in cycling as a result of holding the wrists in a tensed position for too long, so it is important that cyclists adapt their grip occasionally during long rides to avoid fatiguing the joint. Cyclist's palsy (also called handlebar palsy) can result when the ulnar nerve that extends through the wrist to the ring and little fingers becomes irritated. Both carpal tunnel syndrome and cyclist's palsy can be relieved by stretching the hands, fingers, and wrists before riding, and by wearing padded gloves that can help reduce stress to the bones and joints.

Cycling Safety Tips

Cyclists should keep in mind some basic safety guidelines. First, cyclists on the road must travel *with* the flow of traffic. In fact, riding against the flow of traffic is one of the major factors in traumatic cycling injuries. When riding on public roads, cyclists must observe red and green lights, and conform to all traffic rules. Cyclists can use the middle of the lane *only* if they are traveling at the posted speed limit; if they are moving slower than the speed limit, they should generally ride as far to the right side of the lane as is safe. Cyclists must yield the right-of-way at crosswalks to pedestrians. Cyclists who choose to ride on sidewalks should follow all the same rules that pedestrians do, stopping at every corner and crossing with the lights. Unless local laws make a specific exception for cyclists, all motor vehicle traffic laws apply to bicycle riders as well. Make sure that bikes are equipped with red and white reflectors, as well as lamps for evening. Night riding is not recommended. Young cyclists should make sure to always carry sufficient water with them to stay hydrated, as well as a cell phone in case of an emergency. Make sure to discuss with your children which streets are permitted for biking according to the law and your family's own rules, and that they make clear their intended route and how long they expect to be gone before they leave the house.

All told, cycling is an extremely safe sport that can provide an excellent basis for fitness, whether the cyclist is looking to compete or is simply using it as part of a cross-training routine. Simple adjustments to the bike's height and parts, and small fixes to posture or grip, can make a huge difference that will allow riders to stay active mile after mile, year after year.

Chapter 9
Dance

Despite the incredible variety of dance genres—classical ballet, tap, jazz, African jazz, modern, character, crunk, hip-hop, ballroom, Latin, Irish, clogging, Broadway, stomp (just to name a few)—the most common injuries develop consistently in the lower half of the body. As young dancers of all varieties know, hours and hours of practice each week are common. Because of the long hours, injuries related to overuse and extreme body positions are much more likely than injuries due to trauma. Mature dancers are artistic athletes; as a result, young dancers may overuse their bodies in an attempt to achieve this goal. Additionally, the risk of injuries increases as dancers age, so it is of the utmost importance that young dancers learn proper techniques in order to preserve their bodies for future activity.

One of the most fundamental means of combating dance injuries, in addition to proper instruction from a qualified teacher, is a proper warm-up. Since flexibility is key to most dance forms, a thorough warm-up routine is an absolute must before any kind of rehearsing or floor work. Traditional studio dance classes usually open with bar exercises that last anywhere from twenty to forty-five minutes. During this time, an instructor should lay out the warm-up choreography that will not only promote blood flow and muscle movement but will also allow a chance for each dancer's technique to be observed and corrected if necessary.

Body alignment is central to dance, although it may vary based upon the type or the style of movement. For example, classical ballet calls for the leg to be turned out at all times—that is, with the hips, knees, and toes all in alignment. This position is essential for the aesthetic of the dance and provides the most support and safety for the joints. Certain body types can lead to joint motion limitations, particularly with the hip, which can be stressed unnecessarily if the dancer is not supervised properly by a knowledgeable instructor. Other styles incorporate movements that require different postures and body alignment. A qualified teacher can instruct students in the proper form for the kind of dance being studied, and can help the dancer perfect these techniques during the warm-up period.

Dancers should also be aware of how environmental factors may affect their movement. Despite the fact that dance is generally an indoor activity, studios can often be cold or drafty, or performances may take place outside at football games or in parades. Dance costumes are usually designed for their artistic appearance more than for utility; therefore, dancers who are in chilly situations should make sure that they stay in heavier clothes that still allow for movement for as long as possible to retain warmth and muscle elasticity. Also, the dance floor should be taken into account. The oak floor of a traditional studio will absorb shock very differently from concrete or asphalt or athletic mats. This matters when considering leaps, choreographed falls, or other high-impact movements.

Proper shoes are also important. For dance styles such as stomp or hip-hop, sturdier shoes are necessary to absorb the impact of percussive movements or jumps. Similarly, tap shoes or clogging shoes should have properly fitting insoles to protect against blisters or irritation. Pointe shoes in ballet should be used only by female dancers whose skills have been evaluated and approved by a qualified dance teacher who can examine the position of a dancer's foot in the shoe. Premature pointe exposure can cause lasting foot damage, so it's a good idea to consult a podiatrist or a foot and ankle specialist prior to participating.

Perhaps the most potentially dangerous risk for young dancers is one that occurs far from the studio or stage: nutritional deficiencies and, in the most extreme cases, anorexia and bulimia.

For many dance genres, a very lean, slender body is considered the ideal; as a result, many young dancers will purposely deprive their bodies of food in order to achieve this "look." Because it is done for the sake of the art, many dancers, teachers, and even parents fail to see it as harmful and injurious. Nothing could be further from the truth. Good nutrition is especially important during the childhood and adolescent years; nutritional deficits during this time can lead to hormone imbalances, stunted growth, and delays in normal development milestones such as menstruation. Dancers should eat a full, balanced meal three to four hours before a rehearsal or performance and stay hydrated throughout that time. As with any activity, complex carbohydrates such as whole wheat breads and pastas and brown rice are recommended before a particularly long or intense session, coupled with protein to keep the dancer feeling full. Skipping meals or following fad diets is not healthy or wise for growing children and teens.

Dance is one of the main activities in which the female athlete triad is a concern. Parents and teachers alike need to be aware of the issues facing young dancers and be alert to any warning signs that a child may be harboring an unhealthy obsession with weight, whether he or she is drastically altering eating habits or continuing to diet even after shedding the undesired pounds. In some cases, dancers may turn to smoking in order to curb hunger—or even bizarre methods of tricking the body into feeling full, such as swallowing cotton balls to fill the stomach without consuming calories. These unhealthy lifestyle choices are simply not sustainable; improper musculoskeletal development, lung damage, and even a weakening of the heart and other vital organs can occur as a result of anorexia, bulimia, yo-yo dieting, and smoking. The younger a person gets involved in any of these dangerous behaviors, the more difficult it will be to establish positive patterns later.

Dancers and their parents should discuss the various pressures and risks that the dance world brings and determine what alternative steps they should take toward pursuing long-term goals in a healthy manner. Any young dancer who is concerned about his or her weight should meet with a registered dietician or even the school nurse to discuss healthy options for losing or maintaining weight goals. If a dancer feels uncomfortable in dance class attire, he or she should speak with the teacher about other athletic wear options. Finally, if a young person finds that her body type is developing outside the preferred type for the genre, she could explore different dance styles in which fuller-figured or curvier types have a stylistic advantage. Or the dancer could simply decide to prove the detractors wrong and continue in the style she loves for as long as it remains an enjoyable pursuit.

Chapter 10
Equestrian Sports

Horseback riding is among the most popular sports in the world. In the United States, approximately thirty million people participate in equestrian activities every year. These equestrians are drawn together by a love of horses and a sense of freedom that can be felt only while flying on the back of their favorite mount. They enjoy the challenge of conquering high jumps, the adventure of blazing new trails, and the camaraderie of moving as a perfectly harmonized unit with their horse. A passion for horseback riding draws people from all walks of life and causes them to seek out opportunities to ride in a variety of different ways. Rodeos, eventing, dressage, and trail riding are just a few of the many different styles of equestrian participation. Regardless of the type of riding, equestrians must be fearless athletes who persevere through years of hard work to master their sport. They must possess balance, skill, and wise judgment to stay safely mounted on their equine partners.

In the world of sports, horseback riding presents a unique challenge because an essential member of the team is an animal, obviously. Horses have their own temperament and athletic capabilities; they can act independently and sometimes unpredictably. Horses can kick with a force of nearly one ton and can change speed and direction in less than a second. At any given moment, the rider's head may be thirteen feet in the air, traveling at speeds of up to forty miles per hour. Statistics show that horseback riding is more perilous than skiing, automobile racing, football, and rugby. Whereas a motorcyclist can expect a serious incident at the rate of 1 per 7,000 riding hours, a horseman can expect a serious accident once out of every 350 riding hours, making it twenty times more dangerous.

In the United States, more than one hundred thousand horse-related injuries are seen in hospitals every year. Of this number, an estimated twenty-three thousand involve youths under twenty. The severity of these youth horseback-riding injuries is often greater than other sports-related injuries as well. In fact, equestrian riders rank second in number only to pedestrians in being struck by cars, and the injuries from horse-related accidents have a higher severity score than crash injuries involving either all-terrain vehicles, bicycles, or passenger motor vehicles. Most horse-related injuries are sustained when the rider is thrown from the horse, which is often accompanied by being dragged or crushed. However, studies indicate that 20 to 30 percent of equestrian-related trauma occurs while the rider is on the ground. Activities such as leading, grooming, and petting the horse can give a rider a false sense of security. Many riders may not consider a helmet a necessity after dismounting, leaving them vulnerable to kick injuries. Unfortunately, over 50 percent of kick injuries involve the head, neck, or face, and can result in average hospital stays that are nearly three times longer than those from injuries due to falls.

The most common place for horse-related accidents to occur is at sporting venues, followed by the home and on a farm. The most frequent injuries seen are contusions (also called bruises), fractures, sprains, strains, lacerations, internal-organ injuries, and concussions. The most common body parts injured are the head and neck (38 percent), upper extremities (24 percent), and lower extremities (20 percent). Upper extremity injuries are usually sustained when a hand is stretched out to break a fall or when the hand becomes entrapped in ropes, reins, or other horse tack. Lower extremity trauma can occur when the leg is crushed or caught in a stirrup. In total, 11.2 percent of all equestrian injuries will lead to a hospital admission.

Activities with horses also have the potential to be fatal. From 1999 to 2002, there were seventy-six fatal injuries in the United States to youth under twenty years of age. The most frequent cause of death for mounted and dismounted horse activities is head injury. In contrast to the public awareness that was raised after actor Christopher Reeve's spinal accident in 1995, head injuries outnumber spinal injuries by five to one. Unlike in other sports, there are more injuries to the lumbar spine (lower back) and thoracic spine (upper back) than to the cervical spine of the neck.

In equestrian activities, young women are injured more than young men. This prevalence likely reflects the disproportionate number of girls involved in the sport.

Since riding can be dangerous, the cost for managing equestrian injuries is often substantial. Nonfatal injuries treated in the hospital for children under nineteen cost an average of $945.6 million per year.

With personal and monetary costs at stake, it is essential to understand the factors leading to injury and how to prevent them. One of the biggest risk factors for sustaining an injury is the lack of a helmet. Other risk factors are poor judgment, risk taking, poor technique, and poor motor skills. Given the popularity of horseback riding and its potential for injury, physicians should promote strategies to keep riders safe. Helmets should be recommended for all horse-related activities. The helmet should meet the standards of ASTM International (formerly the American Society for Testing and Materials) and should be Safety Equipment Institute (SEI) certified. Although many equestrian sporting events will already have mandatory helmet rules in place, there is no requirement for helmets during rodeos. According to the National High School Rodeo Association, cowboy hats may be worn in lieu of helmets in competition. Even if wearing a helmet, a rider who is thrown should be evaluated carefully for head injury. Concussions are frequent in equestrian sports, and return-to-play guidelines should be similar to those in contact sports. Remember that an athlete need not lose consciousness for a concussion to have occurred and should not return to activity until he or she has been cleared to do so by a qualified health care professional. Please see chapter 31 for more information on concussions.

Appropriate supervision is also critical in equestrian sports. The

American Academy of Pediatrics recommends that young riders be supervised according to their skill level. With the help of an experienced trainer, they should be matched with horses according to their riding abilities. Young horses in the early stages of being broken into saddle and bridle should be avoided until the rider has reached a more advanced level.

Youth riders should also be taught the elements of ground safety. When walking around a horse, children should be trained to respect the danger zones for accidents, namely in front of or behind the horse. They should never wrap ropes or reins around their hands when handling or leading their horses. This practice can result in serious injuries such as finger amputations and shoulder dislocations if the horse pulls away from them.

Safety stirrups may be recommended for young and inexperienced riders. These stirrups have a rubber band that releases when pressure is applied, letting the rider's foot slip out during a fall. This safety measure can prevent a novice from being dragged behind the horse if thrown; it can be a simple way to avoid a life-threatening accident.

Finally, health care providers can prevent horse-related injuries by providing counseling and care to those involved in equestrian events. Patients who have already experienced an injury may be a key target group, because reinjury rates are 25 to 37 percent. Above all, the rider should be treated as a serious athlete. Equestrians participate in a breadth of experiences, ranging from the time-honored traditions of rodeo events and fox hunting to the decorum of the Olympic Games. They must master difficult and dangerous skills with a partner that is unable to communicate using the spoken word. Whether trail riding for pleasure or competing for a national title, a rider takes inherent risks, and injury prevention is essential. Good safety equipment, good technique, and good decision making keep a rider saddled up and safe.

Chapter 11
Field Hockey

Although field hockey in its modern form originated in England in the nineteenth century, its roots actually go back nearly four thousand years. Images of athletes pushing a ball with crooked sticks decorate the tomb walls of the Egyptian pharaoh Kheti. Records indicate that a similar game was played in Ethiopia roughly three thousand years ago. In 1908, men's field hockey became an Olympic sport, but since the game arrived in the United States in 1901, it has been played primarily by women. Women's field hockey finally achieved Olympic recognition at the 1980 games.

Popular at both the college and high school levels, field hockey continues to develop both in terms of numbers as well as in intensity. Even though it is considered a noncontact sport, it still brings the possibility of any number of injuries due to contact with other players, sticks, the ball, or the ground. And unlike its ice-based counterpart, field hockey requires almost no protective gear. Many concerned parents, coaches, players, child advocates, and health care professionals are pushing to change that by providing athletes with additional safety equipment.

The fingers and hands are the most prone to injury in field hockey due to their positioning on the stick. Because the hand consists of twenty-seven bones and very little fat or large muscles to provide a protective layer, it is highly vulnerable to fractures. The simplest and best way to combat hand injury is to wear gloves—the thicker the better, of course (although it is understandable that most players will not want bulky, heavy, hand coverings—especially for games played outdoors in the heat). Gloves designed for and required in lacrosse are a great option for providing some basic protection. Because they are designed for a stick sport, they are thin enough to allow flexibility but are lightly padded in such a way as to absorb some of the impact of a blow to the hand, and may even improve a player's performance by eliminating some of the fear of injury when pursuing the ball aggressively.

And the game does get aggressive. In fact, studies have found that the majority of injuries in field hockey happen within twenty-five yards of the goal, as players engage in fierce tangles and execute strong hits to score or defend. The most serious injuries are to the face. Teeth can get broken when a ball or stick strikes a player in the face. Because mouth guards are recommended but not always required, this is an easily avoidable injury but one that is still far too common. I cannot stress enough the importance of wearing a properly fitting mouth guard. If a permanent tooth is knocked out, you have approximately a one-hour window in which it can be reimplanted safely. The tooth should be located as quickly as possible and handled only by the enameled portion—never by the root. Rinse off any dirt or debris in milk, and keep the tooth wet in either milk, saline, or saliva while it and the injured player are being transported to an emergency dentist.

Other facial injuries include damage to the eyes, either from impact with the ball or stick or from fragments of a broken stick that penetrate the eye socket. If this occurs, the eye should be covered immediately with a patch while awaiting emergency medical attention, provided that there are no foreign objects in the eye. For a penetrating injury, place a disposable cup with the bottom cut out over the protruding object— only a medical professional should attempt to dislodge it—and keep both eyes covered loosely with gauze until emergency medical attention arrives. This is necessary to prevent the protruding object from moving and causing further damage; it also keeps the eye from moving, since both eyes move as a unit.

Goalies stand the highest risk of facial trauma. Goggles are not required but are highly advisable for the position. Recent rule changes by the International Hockey Federation and the NCAA have opened up the door for players to have the option of facial protection equipment; however, the rules do vary from league to league as to what is considered permissible. Players and parents should check on the rules of their own team and push for the option for face masks or goggles if they are not currently allowed by league rules.

Facial fractures can also occur. If a player exhibits swelling or bruising of the cheekbone, nose, or forehead following impact, she should be removed from play immediately and checked for a concussion. If she displays any signs of confusion, disorientation, balance or coordination problems, or speech difficulties, she should be referred to a medical professional right away. Even if no signs of a concussion are present, anyone sustaining a serious blow to the face should not return to the game until she has been cleared by a medical professional. Please see chapter 31 for a more detailed discussion of concussion symptoms, risk factors, and lingering effects.

Leg and ankle protection is also recommended but not required by every league. Although shin guards are not standard gear, I strongly urge players to invest in a pair of soccer shin guards in order to provide the best possible protection for their bones and joints. Knee pads may or may not be allowed according to league rules, so players and parents should be proactive in checking the rules if they wish to use this additional equipment.

The most common injuries that field hockey players will face are ankle sprains. RICE treatment (rest, ice, compression, and elevation) is the best way to treat a sprain; however, if there is bruising visible over the bone, obvious disfiguring of the foot or ankle, or if the pain does not subside within a week or two, consult a physician, as these may be signs of a fracture. Due to the potential for injury to growth plates (see chapter 22 on running), such a consultation is very important if the pain does not subside or the range of motion remains limited.

Because field hockey is a cutting sport with quick changes in direction and momentum, participants are at a higher risk for ACL tears.

If a player feels a *pop* in her knee when she falls or if there is immediate joint swelling, she should be given prompt medical attention. Surgical intervention is required to repair a torn ligament and six months to a year of rehabilitation will be necessary to restore the joint to full working order. The good news is that athletes can almost always return to full participation in the sport they love the next season.

There is also a risk of overuse injuries from field hockey, especially stress fractures in the lower leg and foot due to running. If pain persists after practice or a game, the player should rest until the pain subsides in order to give the bone a chance to repair the hairline cracks. Otherwise she runs the risk of weakening the bone and suffering a much more acute injury. X-rays are not usually able to visualize the fine cracks of a stress fracture; however, if the pain persists or returns with frequency, a doctor may recommend that the athlete undergo a bone scan in the affected area to make sure that the bone has sufficient density to support continued athletic activity. Further diagnostic tests include an MRI or a CT scan.

Lower back pain and tendinitis in the leg and hip are also common because of the posture required by the game. If an athlete feels persistent pain in her back or joints, she should talk to her coach and cease activity until it subsides. A thorough warm-up and gentle stretching exercises can help alleviate some of the pain. The best defense, however, is a preseason conditioning routine that focuses on both flexibility and strength building in three muscle groups: the abdominal core, the quadriceps, and the hip flexors. By gradually adding weight and repetitions, the body will be much more acclimated to the exertion and much more stable when in practice and game situations.

By adopting new policies that will allow for standard safety gear to be optional for players who wish to use it, field hockey will continue to become safer and safer even as it becomes faster and more competitive. Players who prepare for the season wisely and follow all league rules on body contact will be able to enjoy the rush of the sport for years to come.

Chapter 12
Figure Skating

Although skating was both a form of transportation and recreation for centuries in the icy winters of northern Europe, it was not until the middle of the nineteenth century that the aesthetic aspects formalized into a competitive sport. Now each of its four genres (singles, pairs, synchronized, and ice dancing) is among the most popular events at the Winter Olympics. Who hasn't held their breath as they watched a skater launch into the air, spinning like a top, only to land smoothly and effortlessly? There is no doubt that the artistry and athleticism required by figure skating make it a beautiful and impressive sport to watch.

What most spectators don't see (or get a glimpse of only during the "personal interest" segments on TV) are the countless hours spent in rehearsals, perfecting every turn and leap, every lift and jump. Figure skating is, in fact, one of the most time-intensive sports for the athlete and parents alike. As a result, skaters are extremely prone to overuse injuries as they repeat new tricks and routines over and over, resulting in a very high number of stress fractures in the leg and spine.

Young skaters landing from jumps can endure impact up to 100 Gs, or one hundred times the force of gravity, absorbed almost entirely by the lower body. The stress that this places on the leg and lower vertebrae can be dangerous. Once hairline fractures (or tiny cracks in the bone) develop from repeated impact, the structural integrity of the bone is weakened considerably and places the athlete at a much higher risk of acute injury if the condition progresses. If a skater complains of pain after practice, especially in the takeoff leg or the back, he or she should restrict putting pressure on the affected areas until the pain subsides fully. If the pain persists, consult a sports doctor. A temporary break from the sport can pay major dividends in the future by allowing the bone to heal and preventing a severe fracture or debilitating spinal disc damage later.

When mastering new moves, skaters should first practice off the ice with a harness. Only when a jump is mastered on the ground should it be transferred to the ice. This one change in training can save the skater a tremendous amount of impact to the bones and joints of the legs. Skaters should also limit the number of times they repeat a jump in each practice session in order to protect against spine and lower extremity stress fractures. The STOP Sports Injuries organization also recommends that young skaters not attempt to master new jumping or throwing techniques during growth spurts. By holding off for even two weeks when a child is suffering from growing pains, and focusing instead on connecting steps and footwork, a skater can greatly decrease his or her chances of developing a stress fracture. Growth plate injuries, discussed in greater detail in chapter 22, are more likely to occur during growth spurts and can have long-term implications for development and growth. Pay attention to any growing pains a young skater might have, and speak to his or her coach about them. Slight adaptations to the training schedule can have a big impact on the athlete's long-term development.

Another important safety measure is a surprisingly simple one: Check the skates. Not only is it vital to have properly fitting skates, it is also essential that the boot provides sufficient flexibility for a skater to execute moves properly. While it might seem that a stiffer boot would provide more ankle and knee stabilization, an inflexible boot can actually transfer stress to the knee, hip, and back. When shopping for new skates, make sure to look for a boot that will allow for full movement of the ankle—support is still important, but too much rigidity can cause strain on the joints.

The boot itself can also cause irritation and injury in other ways. Simple rubbing from an incorrect fit can cause blisters or, more seriously, malleolar bursitis, in which a fluid-filled sac at the ankle (usually on the interior of the leg) becomes inflamed and swollen. The condition can often be resolved by rest and by using a specialty tool sold at skating shops that slightly alters or "punches out" the shape of the boot in the problem area. In more severe cases, however, the sac may need to be drained by a sports physician and possibly injected with a corticosteroid shot to resolve the swelling.

The opposite problem—that is, too much space in the boot—can bring its own problems. Haglund's deformities (bony bumps on the heel resulting from slippage in the boot) are common among skaters with ill-fitting skates. These bumps can be quite painful and often lead to bursitis as well. This is a common challenge for parents who buy skates a size or two too large in anticipation of a child's foot growing or who want to utilize hand-me-downs from older siblings. Extra padding in the heel or wrapping the ankle can help tighten the fit. "Lace bite" is a rather ominous-sounding condition caused by an improperly fitting boot, wherein the tongue rubs against the ankle and toes, causing pain down the front of the foot. There are several alternatives, including extra padding or an insert that shields the skin from friction. While each of these conditions may seem like fairly minor issues, they have the potential to cause more serious injuries. For example, lace bite can bring about severe irritation to the tendons in front of the ankle to the point of actual rupture. Even something as seemingly insignificant as a blister can cause a skater to modify his or her motions—whether consciously or not—in order to avoid pain or irritation. By altering the proper technique, a skater can land at an incorrect angle or with too much force on a joint or bone, causing a much more serious injury that could have been avoided simply by having taken a few simple precautions.

Most skating injuries are concentrated on the lower half of the body, but the head and shoulders are also at risk. A concussion can result from a jump or throw that was not landed properly. Even if the skater does not lose consciousness, he or she should not return to skating until after being cleared by a medical professional. Signs of a concussion include confusion, disorientation, blurred vision, nausea or vomiting, or trouble with balance or coordination. Please see chapter 31 for more details about immediate and secondary symptoms of concussions.

Dislocated shoulders can also occur from a poorly landed jump or throw. The ice is not forgiving; nor are the boards of the rink. If a properly landed jump can subject the legs to 100 Gs, imagine what landing incorrectly can do to smaller, more fragile bones in the arms. If the athlete has numbness in his or her arm, limited or no movement in the shoulder, or swelling and bruising of the shoulder joint following impact with the ice, dislocation is likely. Examination by a sports physician or other qualified caregiver is necessary to reach a diagnosis, and only a medical professional should attempt to move the bones back into the socket. If the skater appears to be carrying one shoulder higher than the other or there is any kind of deformation in the chest or shoulders, the collarbone may have been fractured, and medical attention is necessary.

The last, and perhaps more important, advice that I can offer is that parents be attuned to their child's emotional state with regard to figure skating. Because so much time and dedication by the athlete and parents are required for proficiency (not to mention all those countless treks to the rink), it is very easy for children to get burned out. This is especially true for athletes enrolled in elite academies. "Professionalism" is a big risk factor for injury and burnout. If your child begins to show reluctance about going to rehearsal or begins to find more and more excuses to miss them all together, it may be time to take a hiatus from the sport. Often, after a month or two, the child will find that he or she misses being on the ice and will be eager to start again with a renewed sense of enthusiasm. Just make sure that you talk with your child about what he is thinking and feeling. Because so much time and money may have already been invested, a skater may be afraid to ask for a break. Make sure your child knows that your love for her has nothing to do with her skating. That support can provide the healthiest possible foundation for all future pursuits, whether on or off the ice.

Chapter 13
Football

Football is one of the most popular sports played by young athletes—and it leads all other sports in the number of yearly injuries. In 2007, more than 920,000 athletes under the age of eighteen were treated in emergency rooms, doctors' offices, and clinics for football-related injuries, according to the US Consumer Product Safety Commission. Some of these injuries are unavoidable, but some can be prevented—or at least minimized—with certain precautions.

Both overuse and traumatic injuries can occur during football due to the combination of intense practice sessions, seasonal weather, high speeds, and full contact. More so than many other sports, football players' bodies are susceptible to collision injuries because of the man-to-man contact involved in blocking and tackling. Despite the use of protective equipment, major injuries such as concussions, spinal injuries, fractures, and knee and shoulder injuries can and do occur on the gridiron with regularity.

Concussion is one of the most serious—and most common—injuries in football, caused by injury to the brain following trauma. While it's obvious that a player is probably suffering from a concussion if he blacks out after a hit, parents and coaches must be aware of the other warning signs as well. Consciousness does not preclude a concussion. If the athlete expresses any change in his mental state, including confusion, amnesia, difficulty concentrating, dizziness, headache, blurred vision, struggling for balance, numbness or tingling, nausea, vomiting, or drowsiness, he should be removed from play immediately and not be allowed to return until he has been cleared by a health care professional. Under no circumstances should the athlete be given NSAIDs or aspirin, as it could lead to further bleeding or swelling. The player absolutely must be pulled from all activity and given immediate medical attention if a concussion is suspected.

The US Centers for Disease Control and Prevention estimates that up to two million student athletes suffer brain injuries each year, and the majority of those stem from football. Teenagers, whose brains are not yet fully developed, are especially at risk for serious damage from concussions. Yet, as any football parent knows, young athletes are often determined to return to the field as quickly as possible—especially on game night. This must be forbidden if the athlete shows any of the indicators of even a mild concussion, such as balance problems or unfocused eyes. Parents and coaches should educate young athletes about the symptoms and dangers of concussions, and emphasize why proper precautions must be taken before play can resume. If the athletes themselves understand the gravity of the situation and its potential long-term repercussions, they can take an active role in their own health.

There is no foolproof way to prevent concussions, although well-maintained and properly fitting helmets and face masks are keys to minimizing the risk of injury. Because of the velocity of the hits, a properly fitting helmet is absolutely the most essential part of a player's uniform. It should fit snugly, covering the ears, forehead, and back of the head. Any cracking or dents should immediately be reported to the coach, and an undamaged helmet should be issued in its place; never play with a helmet that shows signs of distress or fits too loosely. It's always worth investing in a new one in order to protect your brain. Players must also be taught not to tackle leading with the head, as head-to-head contact can lead to traumatic and catastrophic injuries, including concussions, cervical spine injuries, and even death. Youth football referees must be ever cognizant of head-to-head contact and call that penalty aggressively. It is the responsibility of parents and coaches to make sure that referees do their jobs.

The most important thing to remember about spinal injuries is that any athlete with a suspected spinal injury must not be moved in any way except by medical professionals, such as the athletic trainers and paramedics present at most high school football games. If the player has lost consciousness and is not moving, attempting to shake him or move his arms and legs may result in permanent paralysis or even death. Parents should also insist that a fully charged automated external defibrillator is available at the field should a player's heart stop during a game or practice.

Another threat to a player's long-term prospects is his leg health. Perhaps the most famous sports injury in the last fifty years was the comminuted compound fracture that Washington Redskins quarterback Joe Theismann suffered to his right leg playing against the New York Giants in 1985. The gruesome injury, which fractured both the bones in the lower leg, forced Theismann into retirement at thirty-six. The game reel from that moment is a lurid reminder of just how important it is for a player to do everything he can to safeguard his legs in the game.

While some accidents are simply unavoidable, players should still learn how to protect themselves as much as possible. The forces applied to either tackling an opponent or resisting being brought to the ground make football players prone to injury anywhere on the body regardless of protective equipment. The traumatic injuries in football include those to the anterior or perhaps even the posterior cruciate ligament and to the menisci or other cartilage of the knee. Complex knee ligament injuries, such as knee dislocation or tears to the ACL or the medial collateral ligament (MCL), are the most serious. Those injuries can disrupt the arterial supply to the lower extremity. That blood supply has to be repaired surgically in six to eight hours, or loss of limb could occur.

Any of these knee injuries can adversely affect the player's long-term involvement in the sport. Hard surfaces and cutting motions can contribute to ankle sprains, while bracing and twisting can lead to more serious harm to the menisci. Damage to either the anterior or posterior ligament is also a risk. As both cartilage and ligament damage usually require surgical intervention and extensive rehabilitation, it is essential that proper procedures are taken to guard against these injuries as much as possible. As stated above, the most common knee injury in football is the dreaded ACL injury. It can occur from noncontact (60 percent of the time) or from a contact blow. It will almost inevitably require surgery for reconstruction.

Proper stretching is, of course, recommended, as are weight and flexibility training to strengthen the muscles around each joint. Conditioning is also important, as fatigue can contribute to a player's vulnerability to injury. Coaches must emphasize the importance of not locking the knee when blocking. This technique may seem counterintuitive, especially to younger players; however, a joint that is bent slightly and relaxed (the so-called athletic position), even if it is engaged in pushing or bracing, is far more flexible than one that is rigid. If the knee sustains impact while locked, the risk of hyperextension, bone damage, or a dangerous twisting of the joint can result in a very serious injury. Balance exercises, as well as learning to jump and land in a flexed position, are also important preventative measures.

The knees are not the only vulnerable joints; the shoulder joint also sees quite a few injuries from football. Offensive and defensive linemen in particular are susceptible to cartilage injuries in the shoulder socket, which produce dislocations. Athletes should pay special attention to strength training and stretching the shoulders, as well as ensuring that their protective gear fits properly so that the equipment, and not the bone, absorbs the majority of any hit or fall.

Besides traumatic injuries, overuse injuries are also common on the gridiron. Lower back and knee pain can often stem from too much time in the weight room or doing other conditioning activities with an eye toward the amount of weight lifted or repetitions rather than proper technique. A strengthening program focused on the quadriceps is often the most effective use of weight room resources and can also relieve knee pain caused by stressed tendons.

Heat exhaustion can also be a major concern, depending on geography, especially in the summer. If players do not stay well hydrated—which means drinking extra water up to twenty-four hours prior to practice as well as during the workout—they put themselves at risk of cramping and even heatstroke, which can be fatal. If a player begins to feel weak and dizzy, or experience muscle cramps, he should inform a coach or team medical services provider immediately, to make sure that his fluids and salts stay at a healthy level and that the situation does not progress to anything more serious. Weigh-in and weigh-out charts should be mandatory for young football players so that coaches are able to pick up weight changes due to day-to-day dehydration. Parents should make sure that their children are hydrated at home every day. At any sign of heat exhaustion—especially during early-season workouts in the middle of summer—extreme caution should be taken. A rectal temperature of 104 degrees Fahrenheit or higher is to be taken seriously. If a player reaches that critical temperature, there is only about a ten-minute window in which his body temperature can be lowered. Treatment is best done right on the field or in the stadium with ice immersion; if his body reaches 105, heatstroke will set in, triggering failure of the liver, kidney, and other vital organs. Therefore, ice baths and a hydration station *must* be available at all practices.

Staying active during the summer is one of the best ways to start the season on a healthy note and to maintain that level of fitness in every game. Acclimation *before* the beginning of football season is extremely important in combating heat injuries as well as general fatigue and sloppiness in proper form once practices start. The first five or six days of football practice should be one-a-days, not two-a-days, in order to allow for acclimation. Many young athletes today spend most of their early-summer months in air-conditioning, so the heat of August practices immediately zaps their energy unless they are prepared for it.

Additionally, off-season strength training and stretching programs will give a young athlete the best shot at a healthy season. Ballistic exercises (see chapter 32) are very important to really warm up the body prior to football practice; just doing static stretches to warm up is not the best way to prepare. Constantly incorporate strength training and stretching to build muscle and flexibility gradually.

Perhaps the most important advice I can offer, however, is that parents speak with a sports medicine professional or athletic trainer if they have any concerns about injuries or prevention strategies. By opening the lines of communication on the team, everyone can ensure that the child has the best possible playing experiences—which is what it should be all about in the end.

Chapter 14
Golf

Golf is one of the fastest-growing sports among young athletes, for a number of reasons. For one, it is an extremely safe sport in terms of traumatic injuries. It provides a way to stay active and enjoy the outdoors without too much physical stress, which is one of the reasons it can be played by people of all ages. This is why it is also an activity that many families can enjoy together. Golf is also a great source for college athletic scholarships. Many children are starting to golf earlier and earlier in the hopes of reaching elite levels in the game they love.

Unfortunately, as with many youth sports that require long hours of practice, young golfers run the risk of overuse injuries—especially athletes enrolled in golf academies that specialize in one-on-one instruction. While the parents of these golfers believe that they are providing their child with the best possible advantages in mastering the game, they also could be limiting their child's future career inadvertently. I have no objections to private coaching or special developmental courses, but I do want to educate parents on the potential risks and warning signs of detrimental repetition so they can take the best steps to protect their child and maximize his or her potential for success.

The most important way to avoid injury on the fairway is to

develop a technically sound swing. High golf swing velocities can affect the neck, spine, shoulders, elbows, hips, wrists, knees, and ankles. Unfortunately, golf is a unilateral sport, with the right and left sides of the body doing different movements and enduring different forces and stresses. In a right-handed golfer, the left side of the body is injured most often, in particular the left shoulder, wrist, and knee. The opposite is true for left-handed golfers, who tend to see more injuries on the right side of the body. From a statistical standpoint, the lower back is injured most often due to twisting (torsion), compression, and shear loads associated with the golf swing. It is interesting to note that the number one reason for a shortened golf career is chronic lower back problems.

It should be clear that golf can take quite a toll on any part of the body, even if it is considered a low-impact sport. Studies have shown a direct correlation between the rate of injuries and the number of swings executed in tournaments. Since even the slightest variance or adaptive movement can affect a golf swing, a qualified instructor should be employed for anyone just starting out or hoping to improve his or her technique. Almost every golf course has instructors available to help teach the correct grip and movement in each of the four phases of the swing: backswing, downswing, impact zone, and follow-through. Each has its own distinct posture and movement that affect the power and safety of the swing as a whole. An aspiring golfer should always work with a professional to gradually adapt his or her body to the proper form and rhythm of swinging a club before attempting anything other than simple putting.

For the more experienced golfer, the risk of a stress injury due to repetitive motion is a danger. The very first measure I recommend is a thorough warm-up. Although it is a low-impact sport, golf still employs every major joint in the body in one way or another, which means that as tempting as it might be to casually hit the links or the driving range whenever schedule or weather allow, if a golfer's body has not been prepared correctly for the activity, there is a chance that it could sustain injury. A gymnast or baseball player certainly wouldn't twist and swing without first stretching his or her muscles; golfers employ many of the same muscle groups and should make sure to give them the same chance to warm up.

Before hitting a ball, try doing a few trunk twists with your hands on a golf club placed across your shoulders, followed by a few slow swings holding two clubs together, or a weighted club, like a baseball bat. You can even do a set or two of jumping jacks to get the blood pumping, as well as loosen the shoulders. Then focus on stretching the oblique muscles located on right and left sides of the abdomen, as well as stretching the back by touching your toes. See the illustration on page 207 for a suggested stretching routine to maximize warm-up time.

In any warm-up, when beginning to hit balls, start only with a wedge and hit little pitch shots; then move to half-wedges, building slowly to a full swing before progressing to longer clubs—especially a driver. One of the worst things a golfer can do is to start out using a driver to hit as hard as he or she can.

While stretching can reduce the risk of strained muscles and prepare them better for the rigors of exercise, the golfer must also know when to give his or her joints a break. Due to the shoulder's role in swinging a club properly, rotator cuff overuse in the lead shoulder is one of the most common complaints on the fairway. If the shoulder or the side of the neck hurts following a round of golf or practice session, allow the muscles to rest for a day; forcing them to repeat extreme motions while they are fatigued can cause the rotator cuff muscles to develop tendinitis, or even tear and destabilize the shoulder joint. Instead of long drives, work on putting or chipping until the pain subsides. The shoulder is also vulnerable to cramping or stress if the player favors one side or the other while carrying a golf bag. Simply alternating shoulders between holes, or using both shoulder straps if the bag is of that style, can help tremendously in alleviating shoulder pain.

The same is true of the wrist. Any achiness that comes on the heels of swinging the club means that the muscles have been overworked and should be allowed to recover before subjecting the joint to further stress. A conditioning program that targets the shoulder and forearm through light weights and moderate repetitions (between ten and twenty) will help to build up those crucial muscles. Be sure to work the forearm in both the pronated (palm-down) and supinated (palm-up) positions to thoroughly develop all the muscles employed in golf. Carrying a rubber ball to squeeze during the day can be a simple, low-impact way to build up wrist and forearm strength, especially on the weaker side of the body. The upper inner forearm can often become painful when the medial epicondyle is fatigued from your gripping the club too tightly; the condition, often called "golfer's elbow," occurs most frequently in the right elbow for a right-handed golfer and in the left elbow for a left-handed one. It can be combated through a simple, gradual conditioning routine. Always stretch the shoulder, elbow, and wrist after such a workout to make sure that the joints stay flexible. Conversely, lateral epicondylitis on the outside of the elbow can also develop in golf. This is commonly called "tennis elbow" because it is so common on the hitting side of a tennis player. In golf it occurs most commonly on the left elbow for a right-handed player, and vice versa.

Because the core of the body moves so dramatically from one posture to another during the golf swing, it can also become sore if overworked, which can lead to the player adapting his or her swing in potentially harmful ways. The lower back is especially vulnerable, so flexibility and core-strengthening exercises in preseason conditioning can help a young golfer protect his or her body. However, he should pay close attention to what his body is telling him. If the back begins to hurt, it is an indication that something is wrong and the athlete should give the muscles a chance to rest. He or she should address the issue with a golf instructor when the pain has subsided in order to correct any technique that may be off in the swing.

Acute injuries, although rare in golf, can occur. They are usually due to external factors such as the club's striking a rock when playing off the fairway. These injuries can occur in several ways. One cause is from "casting" at the top of the backswing: that is, when the arms raise the club behind the body, preparing to swing downward to strike the ball. If the wrist extends too far, the club may keep moving after the arms have stopped, causing it to veer off in an unintended direction. Another cause can simply be misjudging the landscape and striking the ball at the wrong angle. Either way, if the club head happens to strike a stationary object, the impact will radiate up the shaft and can dislocate the extensor carpi ulnaris tendon of the wrist or fracture one of the wrist bones. Both conditions are extremely painful.

If a golfer is unable to grasp a club or move his or her wrist following unintentional contact with a solid object, seek a medical diagnosis right away. Since the wrist is particularly prone to arthritis in older adults, and since traumatic injury to a joint in youth exponentially increases the risk of arthritis later, this is a serious concern. If the ball happens to land in a particularly precarious setting, young golfers should consider deeming it unplayable. It is essential to remember: The hit their score will take is nothing compared to the impact such an injury could have on their body.

Other external factors that should be taken into consideration are heat and lightning. Anyone wishing to play golf outdoors in the summer should take all necessary precautions against the sun, including headgear and eyeshades and, of course, hydration. To avoid muscle cramps, heat exhaustion, and dehydration, golfers should consume fifteen to twenty ounces of water within an hour of their tee time, as well as bring water with them to stay cooled and hydrated during the round. Golfers should also pay close attention to weather reports and to changing conditions around them. At the first sound of thunder, they should pack up their game and leave the course. If the lightning alarm goes off, suspend play and seek shelter immediately. If no shelter is available, find a low-lying, wooded area clear of any isolated trees and crouch down until the storm passes. Between the trees on courses, metal-spiked shoes in soggy ground, and (of course) metal clubs, the risk of getting struck by lightning is real and serious. Lightning can cause permanent paralysis as well as death. It is no laughing matter. Young golfers must understand that it is never safe to be on the fairway during a storm. If a golfer is struck, call 911 immediately. *Do not touch the body,* as the charge may still be present.

Finally, as tempting as it is to play golf whenever possible, especially for those lucky enough to live in a warm climate, children need time off to allow their bodies to grow, develop, and repair any injuries. Therefore, avoid the temptation to allow young golfers to play year-round.

Designate at least one or two consecutive months each year for the golfer to put aside the clubs and pursue another sport entirely and cross-train, or simply take some time off. This is essential to avoid overuse as well as burnout. Make sure your child's body is protected so that he or she is able to enjoy many more decades of the wonderful game of golf.

Chapter 15

Gymnastics

There is no question that gymnastics is one of the most popular competitive sports, particularly when it comes to attention and interest at the Summer Olympic Games. However, at the grassroots level, gymnastics can be a kind of blanket term that covers a wide variety of physical activity and competition. Although girls' gymnastics programs are far more common in middle schools and high schools, boys' programs are still holding on in many private gyms and also at the collegiate level. One of the major reasons for the difference in popularity among young athletes is tied directly to how each gender matures physically. Girls' bodies tend to develop sooner, and most female Olympic gymnasts are under the age of eighteen. Boys, on the other hand, generally go through puberty later, and their bodies typically reach maximum flexibility and musculature later, too; the average age of male Olympic gymnasts tends to be in the early to midtwenties. Significant, too, are the differences in the types of events: Women's gymnastics has vault, floor exercise, balance beam, and uneven bars, while men's gymnastics consists of vault, floor exercise, pommel horse, still rings, parallel bars, and high bar. Additionally, both rhythmic gymnastics for women and trampolining (also called acrobatic gymnastics) for both sexes have been growing in popularity because of their inclusion in Olympic competition.

Yet despite this wide variance of style, technique, and competitive platforms, the types of potential injuries remain consistent, with the most common injuries involving the lower extremities and usually associated with landings or dismounts. The knee, ankle, and lower back are particularly vulnerable. Who can forget Kerri Strug's incredible finish at the 1996 Atlanta Olympics, landing her second pass on the vault to secure Team USA the gold despite suffering a severe sprain and tendon damage in her ankle? Unfortunately, this type of injury is not uncommon, nor does it generally contribute to so dramatic a happy ending as Strug's.

Each year more than eighty-six thousand gymnastics-related injuries are treated in hospitals, doctors' offices, clinics, and ambulatory surgery centers. Gymnasts must prepare for the rigorous physical and emotional skills that their sport requires. Their hours of gymnastic practice often lead to overuse injuries or even traumatic injuries. If left untreated, these injuries can cause chronic pain, stress fractures, and permanent injuries or pain into adulthood.

When a foot or ankle injury is suspected, the first precaution should be rest and immobilization. If the pain is in the back of the heel, it is likely caused by stress to the Achilles tendon. Gentle stretching in each direction (for example, "writing" the alphabet in the air with the foot) can help restore flexibility and a full range of movement. Achilles tendinitis often causes soreness in the calf muscles as well. Modify activity to address the pain. Avoid jumping or hard landings until the pain has subsided, while working to keep the muscles active and pliable. If the pain persists, it may be necessary for a physician to conduct an ultrasound exam to be sure that the tendon hasn't torn. It is not uncommon even for younger gymnasts to suffer repetitive stress to the Achilles tendon, which is a very serious, career-threatening injury.

Ligament sprains can range from minor to major. A rolled ankle that generates sharp but quickly subsiding pain may need only ice and rest for a few hours to recover. If the pain is isolated to just one side of the joint, it will likely heal within a few days, although stiffness is common.

Treatment is ice compression with rehabilitation to restore function. Once the joint is able to bear weight and the athlete can walk without a limp, activity may be resumed; a brace or taping may be desirable for added reinforcement, however. Should the same joint develop chronic pain or weakness, or become reinjured, it is advisable to consult a sports physician.

An injury that displays bruising and swelling, as well as tenderness to the touch (especially directly over bones) and pain all around the joint, is likely serious. Should this occur, a health care professional should be consulted immediately to determine whether it is a serious sprain or a fracture.

ACL injuries to the knee are commonly associated with gymnastics. These injuries are usually accompanied by a *pop* as the athlete lands on the knee. In gymnastics, this tends to happen by overrotating while tumbling, vaulting, or dismounting from the beam or bars. It can also happen if the gymnast lands short or undercuts a rotation, putting stress on the knee at an unnatural angle. Swelling will accompany an ACL injury and can last for hours or even days. A thorough history and physical exam, along with a routine knee X-ray and confirmatory MRI, are necessary to determine the extent of the injury and, as is the case with other sports, ACL reconstruction may be necessary. Because the injury can be so devastating and the recovery time is extensive (six to twelve months), coaches should always be present as spotters to help ensure that the gymnast has a safe landing until he or she is fully confident in the move and has executed it without incident or assistance (other than the coach's presence) several times in a row.

The upper body has its own set of concerns because it is used to bear weight. Gymnasts who specialize in ring and bar exercises are especially vulnerable to labral tears (also called SLAP tears; an acronym for *superior labrum anterior and posterior*) in the shoulder. These injuries can lead to frank subluxation or dislocation of the shoulder joint. Traumatic falls from gymnastic apparatuses can cause significant injuries to the shoulder also. Dull but throbbing pain that increases with activity is cause for concern. If an athlete complains of consistent shoulder pain and requires regular icing of the joint, it's time for a medical exam.

The elbow and wrist are also subjected to a great deal of force; the wrist is especially susceptible because it often endures forces that regularly exceed double the athlete's body weight. Because this joint is so central to gymnastic activity, special care should be taken to treat any pain symptoms by way of rest, stretching, and bracing. This is especially true if the pain extends to normal movement outside of athletic training. If an injury such as a sprain should occur, the athlete is advised to rest a full six weeks before resuming the sport. One of the more common injuries to the elbow is the so-called OCD (osteochondritis dissecans): a defect of the outer part of the joint, which causes damage to the internal blood vessels in the bone. Due to their wide-open growth plates, prepubescent gymnasts are particularly predisposed. Repetitive strain on the elbow joint can result in a gradual decay of the bone, painful structural defects, and subsequent looseness or locking of the elbow joint. OCD is a career-threatening injury that requires surgical correction.

Lower back pain can be caused by a number of different factors, among them muscle strains, stress fractures, ligament sprains, and disorders involving the intervertebral discs, the gel-like pads that act as cushions between the vertebrae of the spine. Extension movements will tend to aggravate the pain, although any activity can exacerbate it. If the pain is persistent or debilitating, an examination with an MRI or bone scan may be recommended to determine the exact nature of the injury. Pain caused by strains or sprains can usually be resolved through physical therapy and rest.

Finally, parents should make sure that they get to know their child's coach. Because gymnastics can be highly competitive, some coaches have developed a tough-as-nails attitude that can be very damaging for young people. If your child is consistently upset after practice, it may be time to look for a new coach or a new gym entirely. Under no circumstances should a coach ever berate or insult a child; the emotional scars of irresponsible coaching can be just as serious as the physical ones. Always remember that your child's well-being is more important than his or her athletic goals.

While it is impossible to prevent all injuries from occurring, a few commonsense pointers can help to minimize the risk. Many gymnastics injuries can be prevented by the following training guidelines:

1. Wear all required safety gear. Special equipment may include wrist guards, hand grips, footwear, ankle or elbow braces, and pads.

2. Always be fresh and prepared for practice.

3. Make sure that the coaching staff is trained properly and certified in instruction and safety precautions to curtail minor injuries and prevent major ones.

4. Do not play through the pain. Any athlete who is hurt should be evaluated by a sports trainer and, if necessary, a sports medicine physician, and follow instructions for treatment. Gymnasts are very tough athletes and, unfortunately, many of them believe that pain makes them stronger.

5. See to it that first aid is available at all competitions and practices.

6. Remember that treating minor injuries properly can prevent major injuries.

7. Always inspect equipment to ensure that it is in good condition, including the padded floors. Secure mats under every apparatus. Utilize safety harnesses whenever a gymnast is learning a difficult move.

8. Spotters are extremely important in all of these maneuvers. Therefore, insist on spotters, especially when learning new skills but also during routine practice as well as during competition.

9. Warm up muscles with aerobic exercises such as jumping jacks or running in place before beginning training or new activities. These so-called dynamic prepractice performance drills will help to increase blood flow and keep the body flexible as it attempts to master a new technique.

10. Maintain open communication to ensure a shared sense of purpose between you, the athlete, and the coach.

Under the right circumstances, gymnastics can be a wonderful way for children to develop flexibility, fitness, strength, and confidence.

The different skills required for each event can keep a curious or easily bored child occupied in ways that other sports often cannot. The biggest problem in gymnastics is its often highly competitive coaches. As a result, physically vulnerable young athletes are driven to extreme training. By establishing a firm foundation of safety, gymnastics can open the door to a lifetime of healthy activity and a love for the artistry as well as the physicality of sports.

Chapter 16
Hockey

We all know the old joke: "I went to a boxing match, and a hockey game broke out." Unfortunately, hockey has the rather dubious reputation of being a sport of loose teeth and black eyes, flying pucks and flying fists, high-sticking and sucker punches. But many of the associated injury risks have nothing at all to do with the sport's legendary on-ice brawls.

Concussion is one of the most common serious injuries in hockey. Any player whose head makes hard impact with the ice should be removed from play and examined for warning signs; he or she need not have lost consciousness to have sustained a concussion. If the athlete exhibits confusion or disorientation, loss of balance, or simply "not feeling right," he or she should receive further medical attention immediately. Properly fitting helmets can greatly reduce the risk of concussion but do not eliminate it entirely. One advantage for protecting the head and neck that hockey players have over, say, football players is the slickness of the ice. If the body is able to slide when striking the ground, it deflects much of the energy that might have otherwise caused the spine to be jarred or jammed if the body could not move upon impact. Also, the head-to-head contact seen in football is not part of hockey. Even so, concussion remains a serious risk that coaches, parents, and players must all take seriously. See chapter 31 for more information.

Not all impact in hockey occurs from falls on the ice, however. As players are checked into the boards, they run the risk of hurting themselves in a variety of ways. Shoulder injuries are especially common. Dislocations of the shoulder joint and clavicle fractures (broken collarbone) are tremendously painful and greatly reduce range of motion. Dislocated shoulders are particularly common for hockey goalies. If the player is unable to move his or her shoulder or arms following a fall, the joints should never be manually forced to move by another person in an effort to check for injury. This can cause further damage and intensify the player's pain. Swelling, bruising, unsightly lumps under the skin or a sagging shoulder can indicate a broken bone; even if these symptoms are not present, any player sustaining impact to the shoulder or chest who cannot properly move one or both arms afterward should seek immediate medical attention. A dislocated shoulder should be manipulated back into place only by a qualified professional, and will likely require time in a sling to immobilize the joint while the swelling subsides. Remember that the sooner a dislocated joint is reduced (that is, put back into position), the easier the healing process will be.

A broken collarbone will require an X-ray and a cast, sling, or figure-of-eight harness to keep the bone in the proper position for healing. In severe cases, surgery may be required to install plates with screws and/or pins to repair the clavicle. As much as possible, players should try to avoid striking the boards from the side, turning the body instead to the front or back to minimize the direct impact on a joint.

The same is true for protecting the wrists and elbows. Players should use the forearms, not the hands, to brace themselves. This reduces the risk of hyperextending the wrist joint or fracturing its delicate bones, and deflects much of the impact to a stronger part of the arm. Bursitis of the elbow is also a common injury for hockey players. If the bursa (a fluid-filled sac found in all joints) becomes inflamed or irritated due to repeated stress from falls, it can swell, cause pain similar to bone chips, and limit motion. Repeated strikes can cause scarring and thickening of the bursa, which may necessitate a draining or even an open surgical excision. Elbow pads with a hard outer shell and cushioned interior provide the best protection against this condition, as well as rest and anti-inflammatory medications such as over-the-counter NSAIDs, as soon as pain is detected.

The hip is also susceptible to bursitis following repeated impact with the ice or boards, but this can be reduced by hockey pants with extra padding at the joints. Hip strain is also a common problem that is best treated with rest and best prevented by preseason conditioning of the hip flexor muscles, which can improve flexibility and strengthen the joint. Pulled muscles in the groin can also occur due to skating maneuvers or sliding on the ice. Proper stretching before the game and "cool down" stretching following it can help to build flexibility and reduce strain.

Knee injuries, such as ACL damage and meniscus tears (torn cartilage in the knee), are also common due to the body-to-body contact of the sport, which is further complicated by the inclusion of sticks. Not only does the athlete run the risk of getting tangled in a mass of arms and legs as the players all vie for the puck, but he or she also must try to avoid getting caught around the sticks in the melee. Leg sprains, particularly the medial collateral ligament (MCL) of the knee, sometimes occur when players push off the inside of the skate for acceleration. If there is a popping sensation in the knee or leg, or a sudden sharp pain from a joint wrenching, the player should leave the game immediately. A sprain will require several weeks of active rest and perhaps bracing, while an ACL or meniscus tear almost always requires surgery and extensive rehabilitation. Knee pads or braces can help athletes reduce their chances of injuring the leg but certainly cannot eliminate the risk. Players should learn to move with the twisting of their joints in a pileup rather than tensing the muscles and resisting the movement, which can cause further damage and tearing. Flexibility exercises and mental workouts to stay calm and loose under high-pressure situations will have a major impact on a young athlete's ability to protect his or her body from injury. Increased flexibility in the pelvis, especially the hip flexor muscles, will also help reduce lower back pain. Strengthening the core muscles can also help alleviate stress to the abdominal area. When players lean forward to move the puck, the muscles of the lower back are held in a flexed position and can fatigue or suffer strain if not stretched sufficiently prior to play.

Another all-too-common injury in hockey is tooth loss. Although mouthpieces are mandatory in games, some athletes choose not to wear them during practice or casual play. Make sure that your child is never without his or her mouth guard, as it provides the best possible form of protection. In the event that a tooth is knocked out, however, the treatment will vary depending on the age of the athlete. If it is a baby tooth, parents should contact their dentist immediately, and under no circumstances should they attempt to reinsert the tooth, as this could damage the tooth bud of the adult tooth underneath. If the damaged tooth is permanent, it is critical that the athlete be seen by a dentist within one hour of the injury. The tooth should be handled by the enamel and not by the root, and should be cleaned in milk and then stored in either milk or saline while being transported for emergency medical attention. If the tooth is allowed to dry too much, its ability to be replanted successfully within that crucial one-hour window is reduced.

Finally, no discussion of hockey injuries would be complete without a look at black eyes, lacerations, and bloody noses. Eye injuries can occur following any kind of injury to the center of the face, including the nose and cheekbone, not just the eye socket. Every time a player is struck in the head or face, your immediate concern must be concussion. If there is any fluid coming from the eye, blood visible on the eye, cuts around the eye area, or vision changes (including a loss of vision, blurriness, or seeing double), seek medical attention immediately. An emergency room staff can determine if the injury is confined to the eye (in which case the player may be sent to an ophthalmologist) or if there is an additional injury, such as a facial fracture. If the player is conscious and has a foreign object, such as part of a broken stick, protruding from the eye, punch out the bottom of a paper or Styrofoam cup and place it over the foreign item so that it is not disturbed during transport. Cover *both* eyes (since they move as a unit) and seek medical attention immediately. If the player is unconscious in such a situation, do not attempt to move him in case there is injury to the spinal cord. Only emergency personnel should move the player. Lacerations, especially those about the face, need to be seen quickly in an emergency room or by the team physician for cleaning and suturing.

If no serious injury has occurred to the eye, the player should ice the affected area. Like any other bruise, when the blood vessels are broken, fluid will pool under the skin; because the area under the eye is soft and fatty, it tends to hold this fluid. The slightly transparent nature of the skin often causes it to bruise noticeably. Athletes should be prepared to sport a shiner for a few days. (Most hockey players will be just fine with that. It's called a "battle scar"!)

Nose injuries are also a concern. If a player has a bloody nose, he should keep his head elevated but should not tip his head backward in an attempt to stem the blood flow, as this can cause choking. Instead, he should gently pinch his nose just below the bridge, where the cartilage meets the bone. If the bleeding, bruising, or swelling is severe, or if vision is affected, medical attention is necessary. Additionally, if there is internal swelling or misalignment that does not seem to be healing after a few days and causes a disruption to normal breathing or sleeping, the athlete should consult an otolaryngologist (ear, nose, and throat specialist). If there is an obvious exterior nasal deformity, the sooner it is reduced by a specialist, the better.

Hockey is a tough sport with tough players, but they should know that playing through pain will not make them better players—it will only make them more vulnerable to further injuries that can limit their playing time or even end their career. By practicing and playing safely, players can enjoy many years on the ice (or in the penalty box).

Chapter 17
In-Line Skating and Skateboarding

Skateboarding rose to prominence as part of the teenage culture in America in the late 1970s. A major drought and a recession hit California simultaneously, leaving many cement canals and swimming pools dry. Intrepid young athletes realized that the sloping sides of these empty spaces looked an awful lot like the shape of waves in the ocean, and that a board on wheels might mimic the motion of surfing. And so skateboarding began. What started out as a counterculture form of rebellion has now become an extremely popular mainstream sport, with an active lobby trying to get it introduced into the Olympics. Celebrity skateboarders like Tony Hawk have even become household names. The balance, strength, and discipline required to master both speed and tricks on a skateboard are just as grueling as training for any other sport, and the advances in safety equipment and training techniques have made it far safer in recent years.

In-line skating, a similar sport that began in a very different climate, started as a way for hockey players to stay conditioned when they were away from the rink. In-line skating first gained popularity in the upper Midwest, and by the early 1990s, it was a nationwide phenomenon. Today it continues to attract fans who love racing, powerblading, freestyle slalom skating, or just getting a solid workout. In fact, in-line skating is a highly effective, low-impact way to burn a lot of calories without adding additional stress to the lower extremities. For this reason, athletes suffering from shin splints or other overuse injuries often turn to in-line skating to prevent their muscles from atrophying while they recover.

But whether a young skater is using a board or skates, the same precautions should be taken to protect joints and bones. Overuse injuries are generally not a concern in skating; although muscle fatigue may set in after a long or intense practice, the more serious concern is traumatic injuries; namely, fractures, sprains, and abrasions. And, as you will quickly see, the main thing I will be discussing in this chapter is safety gear, safety gear, *safety gear*! Helmets are always advisable, but protection for the rest of the body is important as well. Some studies have shown that wrist guards can reduce the number of injuries by up to 87 percent, elbow pads by 82 percent, and knee pads by 32 percent.

Without a doubt, the wrist is the most vulnerable joint for any skater, as it becomes the body's natural means of bracing the body against a fall. The impact of hitting the ground or half-pipe can break any of the several small bones in the wrist. If you suspect a fracture, call a doctor. Studies have shown that fractures compromise approximately two-thirds of all serious wrist injuries in skating. Sprains are common too, as are scrapes along the wrist and the ball of the hand if a skater falls and slides. In all cases, wrist guards can help protect the joint, skin, and delicate bones of the hand. Look for wrist guards that fit snugly without restricting blood flow to the fingers and that provide extra padding where the palm of the hand meets the wrist, as this is the area that generally endures the most stress. While some skaters will insist that extra gear restricts motion and makes tricks more difficult to execute, skaters of all levels, even advanced skaters, should wear wrist guards at all times. A wrist guard is far less restrictive than a cast or a surgically repaired wrist with metal plates and screws to hold it together.

Helmets are also extremely important and should never be considered optional. Any skater with dreams of competing in the X Games should be aware that helmets are required in competition. A good helmet should fit securely and contain a slick outer shell that will slide easily on any surface. This feature will help to deflect the energy of a fall at a high speed, and prevent the head from catching on the ground and jarring the vertebrae of the neck. The challenge, of course, is that in-line skating and skateboarding are often practiced independent of coach or adult supervision. Therefore, it is important for young skaters to know the warning signs of a concussion and know when to call a parent or other responsible adult to take a hurt skater for medical evaluation. Even if a skater does not black out, it is still possible that a mild traumatic brain injury could have occurred due to the impact of the brain being forcibly shaken against the inside of the skull. If a fellow skater seems at all confused, dizzy, nauseated, physically unbalanced, or complains of a headache after hitting his or her head, alert an adult immediately and do not resume activity until help arrives. Never allow the injured person to take aspirin, which can worsen the condition by causing further bleeding. Parents must also be made aware of any head injuries or potential concussions that may have occurred so that they can monitor their child for sleeplessness, restlessness, or other uncharacteristic behavior. These symptoms may last up to three weeks after the accident. If a skater exhibits any of these symptoms, consult a medical professional at once. Concussions, like any brain injury, can pose long-term health risks if left untreated. See chapter 31 for further details.

Elbow pads and knee pads with hard plastic casings over the joints are also important safety gear for skaters. If a skater loses control and falls backward, the elbows will almost certainly receive the brunt of the impact. A protective shell can prevent the bones from cracking or chipping and the skin from splitting. In the event of a fall, knee pads can also protect against cracks or bruises to the kneecap and its surrounding ligaments and tendons. While it is hard to predict exactly how a skater may fall, due to the wide variance in speed, angle, momentum, and surfaces on which he or she may be attempting to race or perform a trick, well-fitting gear in good condition can at least provide some form of protection against traumatic injury.

Anyone who is new to wheeled skating sports should begin with lessons, which are often offered at local recreation centers, skating supply shops, and even school clubs. It is important that aspiring skaters learn about proper form, control, and how to use the skates' brakes properly, as well as how to evaluate safe skating conditions to avoid traffic or surfaces that may cause falls. Skaters should also learn about their equipment: how different board lengths can affect the way a skateboard is maneuvered, how differing numbers of wheels in in-line skates can affect speed and movement, and how to keep everything in proper repair. Most importantly, these classes can help athletes develop their skills in a controlled and supervised environment appropriate to their ability. Many accidents occur when novice skaters attempt unsupervised tricks beyond their skill level.

Skating is an exciting, dynamic sport that continues to grow in popularity, both competitively and recreationally. It's your job, as a parent, to ensure your child's safety on the blacktop or the half-pipe. As with any extreme sport, the thrills are as high as the risks. Be careful, supervise your kids, and *good luck*!

Chapter 18
Lacrosse

Lacrosse is one rough sport. Even in girls' leagues, which are generally not full contact, the aggressive nature of chasing the ball, hurling it across the field, and blocking with the body or stick means that this game is not for the faint of heart. But lacrosse is also a sport requiring an incredible amount of finesse, skill, and delicate movement, and as a result, the injuries can range from blunt force trauma to joint stress. In order to help an athlete reach his or her maximum level of performance, parents must have a thorough understanding of the rules as well as the different types of training required by the sport.

First, it's important to recognize the differences in the rules of the game for each gender. Although they are generally alike, there are some significantly different regulations for boys and girls regarding physical movement and protective equipment.

Boys' lacrosse tends to be very high impact. As a result, helmets with full face guards must be worn at all times, including at practice. Given the high impact and potential for stick tangles, the risks of falls and concussions are quite high. The speed with which the ball is flung also necessitates a mouthpiece and goggles. Athletic cups made of hard plastic should be worn, as with any impact sport. Shoulder pads and thickly padded gloves are also a must to protect the collarbone and the hands. Elbow pads, while not required, are also highly recommended, as an elbow injury can limit range of motion for the rest of the child's life. It can also pose a threat to the growth plates in the arm, stunting or even deforming bone development. (For a more detailed discussion, see chapter 22.)

Girls' lacrosse has less mandatory equipment: Only protective goggles and mouthpieces are required. Even though other articles are optional, however, this does not mean they should not be worn. Soft headgear, for example, can help protect the skull from impact. Knee pads, elbow pads, and lightweight gloves can also help deflect the impact of a fall and prevent abrasions and bruises.

In fact, bruises rank among the top health risks for both boys' and girls' lacrosse. Perhaps they don't sound like a big concern, but bruises are often the result of a much more serious injury than simply broken capillaries. Even a moderate bruise can indicate further bleeding under the skin, and the accumulated fluid can form a hard lump that may actually restrict circulation to the surrounding tissues. This is especially dangerous in the head and neck, as well as around joints.

Additionally, strains and sprains are common among lacrosse players. Cutting and dodging, which are so crucial to the game, can often result in muscle strains of the hamstrings, quadriceps, and groin. These noncontact injuries are common among both boys and girls. Ligament sprains to both the knee and the ankle are of special concern. Studies have shown that ankle sprains represent roughly 21 percent of all reported injuries for girls and 16 percent for boys at the scholastic level. The best treatment for a sprain involves RICE therapy (rest, ice, compression, elevation). Any player nursing a sprained ankle should stay off of it for at least a week or two (depending on severity) before reintroducing stretching and movement. If sharp pain, swelling, or bruising persists beyond two weeks, there may be a more serious problem, such as an undetected fracture to the ankle or to one of the delicate bones of the foot. Under these circumstances, you should consult a physician.

Even though ankle sprains are the most common injury for lacrosse players, knee injuries rank as the number one cause of lost playing time. If a player feels a *pop* or tear in his or her knee, and the leg can no longer support weight, an anterior cruciate ligament (ACL) tear is the likely culprit. Unfortunately, the only treatment is surgical repair, with a recovery and rehabilitation time of around six to twelve months. The good news, however, is that athletes who must undergo the surgery are almost always ready to play again by next year's season provided that they have followed a safe rehabilitation plan. I would remind parents and young players alike how important rehabilitation is. As a matter of fact, rehabilitation is often more important than the actual surgical procedure itself.

Although ACL tears are not 100 percent preventable, athletes can take some steps to protect themselves. A comprehensive preseason workout routine that aims to enhance strength and flexibility in the quadriceps and calves will help the muscles form a natural brace around the joint to keep it stable, while also allowing it some stretch and movement if it is suddenly torqued at an unnatural angle. Players should always warm up properly before practices and games, making sure that their joints are limber before taking the field. Ten to fifteen minutes spent stretching each major muscle group thoroughly can save months of physical therapy. Lacrosse players should also strive for greater body awareness, always being mindful of how they are turning and stretching in play and avoiding sudden twists or jerks that will pull a joint into an unnatural position. Balance exercises, such as rolling balance boards, can help players learn how to keep their knees bent in the athletic posture when looking to pass, which can also help to prevent tearing ligaments.

Head and face injury, including concussion, are less common but still a concern in lacrosse. For boys, the most frequent causes are related to physical contact with another player or with the ground; for girls, head injuries are more likely to result from another stick or the ball itself. The importance of helmets and protective eyewear cannot be stressed enough. If a player is struck in the face with a ball, make sure that his or her vision is not disrupted and that there is no blood visible on the eyeball. If the eye seems to have sustained damage, or if there is severe swelling, bruising, or bleeding on the face or head, seek medical attention right away. See chapter 16 for a more detailed examination of how to properly treat eye and nose injuries.

Being struck with the ball can also result in commotio cordis, a disruption of the heart's regular rhythm. Most common in baseball and hockey, commotio cordis does present risks in lacrosse as well. If a ball or a puck strikes the chest at a high rate of speed, it can trigger cardiac arrhythmia, which is an irregular rhythm of the heart. The condition is best treated by early activation of emergency medical services (EMS) and utilization of an on-field automated external defibrillator (AED). Tragically, in February 2012, a twelve-year-old boy died as a result of being hit in the chest with a lacrosse ball. He was reportedly wearing all required safety equipment, which is why the presence of AEDs on the sidelines (and individuals trained and qualified to use them properly) is especially important. Some accidents are simply unavoidable, and we must make sure we are prepared to give every young athlete the best possible chance for recovery should the unimaginable happen.

The best advice for parents is to educate themselves on the level of contact, types of hits, and which elements of safety equipment are permitted in their child's league. They should also avoid tampering with protective equipment beyond basic fit issues, as modifications can compromise the gear's protective qualities. Despite the temptation to use hand-me-down equipment for both convenience and economy, parents should do so only if the fit is proper and the items are not previously damaged. Protective equipment that is too large or too small provides only nominal protection, and can contribute to sloppy play and blisters.

For the athletes themselves, it helps to maintain a basic level of cardiovascular fitness year-round; in the weeks leading up to the start of the season, the emphasis should shift toward more specialized training. Plyometric exercises that emphasize developing fast-twitch muscles should increase gradually. Explosive movements and start-and-stop exercises are essential for the sudden shifts in momentum and energy during game play. Starting with interval running (slower paced jogs punctuated with shorter segments of all-out sprinting at roughly a 3-to-1 ratio) can be a good transition to fast-twitch muscle training, which focuses on sudden bursts of speed, muscle movement, or flexibility.

Beginning with a proper warm-up, which is especially important in plyometrics, will not only help to protect the muscles and tendons from damage but also increase the efficiency of the workout by increasing blood flow. It is essential that such conditioning be undertaken only by an athlete already in good physical condition and under the supervision of a qualified coach or trainer, because the risk of injury is higher in this sort of workout than in basic cardiovascular exercise. The athlete should be completely injury free before undertaking plyometrics in order to avoid adaptive movement—that is, slight modifications to posture, gait, or range of motion in order to compensate for pain. Because the movements are so focused and intense, even an otherwise minor injury could lead to incorrect form, which might damage another joint or muscle during training, or could cause faulty or incorrect muscle memory and contribute to long-term damage.

Additionally, overuse injuries can be a concern in lacrosse. Players should have, at minimum, one to two days off per week. As difficult as it may be to convince most die-hard lacrosse players to put down their sticks, players should also take off at least a month or two each year in order to prevent training fatigue and burnout. A well-rested athlete will hit the field with a renewed love for the game, and this can greatly increase physical and mental performance for the next season.

Lacrosse is one of the most rapidly growing sports in our country. It goes without saying that safety is of the utmost concern, and I hope that all the young men and women who are practicing the sport or even just discovering it for the first time will embrace these suggestions for a healthy and long lacrosse career.

Chapter 19

Martial Arts

Martial arts can be one of the best options for young people who are just beginning to become physically active, because it begins with low-impact training, stresses mental and physical discipline, and requires proficiency before you advance to the next step. It is also one of the fastest-growing sports in the United States, with approximately eight million participants. I read recently that judo is poised to become the most-practiced sport in the world after soccer. On a personal note, my wife and two of my daughters are involved with martial arts; one of my daughters even discussed it with her husband and her ob-gyn and received the thumbs-up to continue with it during most of her pregnancy because it is more about individual movement, stretching, and discipline than about contact. In fact, many martial arts schools do not even permit students to have any physical contact with another person in the degree levels; therefore, only when a student has demonstrated a certain level of skill and discipline may he or she progress from studying stances and techniques to actually executing moves or having body-contact with an opponent.

One of the main reasons for the broad appeal of martial arts is that every branch provides tremendous opportunities, from beginners' classes to highly skilled levels, meaning that it can be practiced and enjoyed by people across the spectrum of talent, fitness, and dedication. It also is a tremendous means of building self-confidence and a sense of security because of the self-defense applications. For this reason, various forms of martial arts are popular choices for young women preparing to move away from home for the first time, as well as for younger children facing physically threatening bullies at school. And the options are tremendous. Adapted capoeira movements (Brazilian dance-fighting) are growing as a popular form of cardio training with a practical self-defense application, so practitioners can pursue fitness while also learning how to fend off would-be attackers. Some classes offer a specific form of martial arts, such as Krav Maga (defensive street fighting developed by the Israeli army); other times, classes just teach a variety of effective techniques taken from several different styles in a kind of crash course in simple but highly effective defensive moves. Even if the techniques are never employed for self-defense (which is clearly the hope), there are tremendous peace of mind and empowerment that come from knowing that you have the means of protecting yourself.

Because of the wide array of martial arts genres, it can be both exciting and a little overwhelming to select one to study. The culture and history of each lends it a distinct style, from Japanese to Korean to Brazilian to Israeli, to combinations of all these and more. As a result, the injuries stemming from each branch can vary; for example, styles that emphasize throwing the opponent (such as judo or aikido) or that put an emphasis on striking blows (such as the Thai combat sport muay Thai and kickboxing) have a naturally higher risk of injury.

However, under well-supervised practice conditions, severe injuries are quite rare. The most common mishaps are minor cuts and bruises to the hand and foot. In karate, if a kick or strike is executed improperly or is blocked, the attacker's body part that absorbed rather than deflected the majority of the blow may suffer some pain from broken capillaries beneath the skin or from a split in the skin itself. If this occurs, the participant should quickly clean up the blood, place a bandage over the cut, and wait until the stinging subsides before continuing. Unless there is significant pain, joint immobility, or sudden swelling, the injury is not likely to be severe. In martial arts where joint locking is employed, such as the Korean practice of Kuk Sool Won, there is a risk of fracture or dislocation. Under professional supervision and instruction, this is rarely a concern. If a more serious injury to the bone or joint is suspected, however, because of severe pain, bruising over the bone, or a visual deformity of the bone after impact, medical attention should be pursued.

Some forms of martial arts, such as jujitsu, Kuk Sool Won, and Kali Silat (an art from the Philippines), employ choking as part of their defense techniques. In such cases, it is possible that a person could lose consciousness or suffer a neck injury. This is yet further reason why a certified, professional instructor is absolutely necessary to oversee training sessions. If an athlete does lose consciousness while practicing one of these moves, he or she should not resume activity after waking if there is evidence of any pain, confusion, or dizziness. If a neck injury is suspected and the athlete cannot move, medical emergency personnel should be summoned immediately. Do not attempt to move the injured person, as this could cause damage to the spine. Wait for a certified medical team to arrive with the proper bracing and support boards to transfer the injured person for further evaluation and care. Emergency medical technicians (EMTs) are well trained in this type of emergency.

Many forms of martial arts use weaponry, although in the United States, these are less common than bare-handed techniques and certainly less common among children and teenagers. Unlike the most popular arts that employ only the body and require very little or no protective gear, protection is absolutely essential when studying knife work, fencing, or other swordplay. Even if stylized rather than authentic weaponry is used (such as the bamboo swords now used in kendo in place of traditional steel blades), properly fitting protective equipment should still be worn on the head, hands, chest, and abdomen. Any qualified teacher will make sure that such items are provided and that all proper safety precautions are taken before beginning instruction.

One last precaution to consider is that in many martial arts competitions, participants are judged according to weight class. Since there is an obvious advantage to being at the high end of a lower weight class than at the low end of a higher one, athletes will sometimes try to drop a few extra pounds before a competition to "make weight." This can contribute to the female athlete triad, when a young woman practicing martial arts becomes obsessed with reducing her weight and adopts unhealthy dietary habits as a result. This can also lead some competitors to attempt drastic means for quick weight purging, such as forgoing all fluids for twenty-four hours, taking laxatives or vomiting to rid the body of food, or attempting to sweat out excess water weight through the use of steam rooms or saunas. Parents and instructors should pay careful attention to a child's eating habits and behaviors, especially leading up to a competition. While it may be natural for an athlete to cut back on portions a day or two ahead of a match, nutritious meals are still important to fuel and sustain the body; food should never be eliminated completely. If an athlete seems lethargic, irritable, shaky, or has heart palpitations, his or her blood sugar may be too low as a result of insufficient nutrition. Fruit juice and complex carbohydrates such as bread or crackers can quickly bring blood sugar levels back to normal, though it may take several hours for the child to fully regain strength.

Again, I cannot emphasize enough the importance of working only with a properly trained and certified instructor. Children should never practice strikes, kicks, or other contact without the supervision of their instructor; nor should they pursue unhealthy and potentially dangerous diet habits. Ask about the credentials of teachers at your local martial arts center; most places are happy to share the qualifications and experience of the instructors they employ. If you feel that a class is too wild or unrestrained in terms of physical contact, speak to the instructor afterward about your concerns. Feel free to ask questions about the types of martial arts taught there and work with the staff to find the style that seems like the best match for your child, depending on your goals: physical fitness, self-defense, self-confidence, and so on. Remember that discipline and control are at the heart of all martial arts.

I've found that the various forms of martial arts provide a rigorous and strenuous workout as a safe and productive way to maintain fitness for young and old alike.

Chapter 20
Rowing

Thanks to Title IX, rowing has been growing in popularity as a traditionally male sport that now has a high number of female participants as well. (We will be discussing Title IX in greater detail in chapter 34.) While rowing is practiced mostly at the college level, it is gaining headway in high schools too and well outside its traditional geographical boundaries of the Northeast.

Rowing requires a tremendous time commitment, however, as it is much more involved than simply going to the school gym or the adjacent practice fields. Rowers must actually travel to the local lake, river, or beach where the boat is docked. It also is a team sport in a very different manner than traditional team sports; rather than each athlete manning his or her own position and moving independently during competition, the rowers work as a unit. For this reason alone, it is an incredible team-building activity.

Each racing competition, including time trials, stake racing, side-by-side racing, and endurance matches, has its own devotees; but side-by-side racing has become especially popular because it is the method used in the Olympics. Besides the format of the competition, the main difference in rowing styles comes down to its two distinct types: sweeping and sculling. Sweeping involves rowers positioned in pairs on either side of the boat, each with both hands on one oar. Sculling places the rowers in a line, one behind the other, each holding two oars. Although the style and finer points of technique for each type differ, the basic anatomy of a stroke is the same. The "catch" is the moment before the oar hits the water, and the "extraction" is the movement of the oar through and out of the water. As the oar enters the water, the rower extends his or her legs, pushing the body toward the bow (front); when the legs are fully extended, the torso is bent toward the bow and the arms are brought up to the chest as the rower straightens the torso again. Good posture efficiently captures the most energy from the muscle movements and transfers them to the oars as they propel the boat through the water. A rower with habitually rounded or hunched shoulders will expend far more energy with far less power, causing quick fatigue and very little motion.

Because of the cyclical nature of these movements repeated continually throughout a race, almost all injuries in rowing are tied directly to overuse, and the same joints in the wrist and the knees tend to bear the brunt of the fatigue. Overuse injuries in rowing are aggravated by colder temperatures, so one of the simplest precautions is to wear warm clothing that protects the vulnerable joints from exposure to the cold air. It is even advisable to seek extra-long sleeves that extend over the wrist, hand, and top of the oar so as to preserve body heat and keep the joint moving more freely.

Overuse injuries in the wrist often take the form of extensor tenosynovitis, which can best be compared to a severe case of writer's cramp—that is, the joint develops crepitus (a creaking sensation) when bent, and pain or a slight swelling is exacerbated by movement. Cock-up splints, commonly used for carpal tunnel syndrome, hold the hand and wrist in a rigid "cocked-up" position that limits unnecessary movement and allows the tendons, ligaments, and muscles to recover after a high-intensity workout. Of course, with any inflexible splint, the wearer runs the risk of atrophy if he or she keeps the joint dormant for too long. Most rowers with wrist pain, however, find that wearing a cock-up for a short time helps to alleviate the pain.

Patellofemoral pain, or pain around the kneecap, is similar in nature to wrist pain in rowing. There may be irritation and some swelling, but the most telltale sign is usually a creaking or clicking when repeatedly bending the knee joint beyond 90 degrees, such as when rowing, doing leg presses or squats in a conditioning program, or climbing stairs. While a knee brace may help to minimize harmful movement, proper stretching is a more permanent solution to help reduce the pain. A second issue facing rowers is iliotibial band syndrome, wherein friction from the band's continual rubbing on bone may lead to a thickening of tissue extending from the thigh to the knee, causing the knee to sting. This condition tends to intensify when the foot strikes the ground or when the knee is subjected repeatedly to a great deal of flexing and extending. While rest, ice, anti-inflammatory medication, and stretching may be enough to relieve the irritation, it may be necessary to undergo an ultrasound scan to determine the extent of the thickening and to rule out any other knee issues.

The trunk of the body also experiences its share of pain when overused in rowing. Lower back pain due to a disc injury is extremely common, and often is aggravated when the student must sit still in class for extended periods of time following practice. The pain may spread through the buttocks and down one or both legs, causing discomfort at best and a great deal of pain and even back spasms at worst. If injury to one of the spinal discs is suspected, the athlete should suspend his or her rowing and weight conditioning to focus instead on stretching and core stabilization exercises. Only when the pain has subsided and the back and abdominal muscles have been strengthened should the athlete ease back into rowing and weight lifting, although adaptive exercises for flexibility and core strength should be retained as part of regular training sessions to prevent relapse.

Stress fractures of the ribs are also preventable by core and flexibility training. This injury usually begins as a dull pain in the chest while the rower is strength training with heavy weights. If the action is continued, the pain will usually progress around the chest to the side and back. It is often accompanied by a worsening cough and discomfort while lying down. Stress fractures in the ribs tend to occur during winter training, so many athletes write off the symptoms as a cold or other seasonal ailment. Additionally, X-rays are not usually able to pick up the thin lines of the fracture, which can further complicate diagnosis. A bone scan is therefore the most reliable way to identify a stress fracture. If a stress fracture is confirmed—or even just suspected—all athletic activity should cease immediately. Once the athlete has healed sufficiently, and the pain is no longer present during normal day-to-day activities, he or she can ease back into training, starting with cycling to rebuild cardio fitness, and then progressing to ergometer training at minimal resistance to measure and control the amount of work performed.

Although it is often difficult for rowers to tear themselves away from their sport, since it means leaving the water entirely, it is essential that they understand the long-term impact of their injury on the team's performance. A short time away from the boat while recuperating can make a world of difference in terms of comfort, ability, and contributing to the team's success when the injured rower returns healthy and ready to row.

Chapter 21
Rugby

According to a British expression, "Football is a game for gentlemen played by thugs, whereas rugby is a game for thugs played by gentlemen." While variations on the game date back to Bronze Age Britain, as well as to ancient Greece, the first formal rules of play were written by the Rugby School in Britain in 1870. As popular as rugby is in such far-flung places as Scotland, Ireland, South Africa, Australia, New Zealand, Canada, France, and throughout South America, it has historically struggled to gain a wide-spread foothold in the United States. Ironically, in both 1920 and 1924, the American rugby team won Olympic gold; however, the sport was dropped from the Games in 1928. But a vote on October 12, 2009, reinstated rugby, which will return to the 2016 games in Rio de Janeiro, Brazil—and the United States will play to defend its ninety-two-year title as the reigning Olympic champions.

Formerly known mostly to northeastern prep schools, rugby has experienced a recent surge in popularity, with new teams and leagues popping up across the country. From charter schools in urban Washington, DC, to colleges in California (and clubs in just about every state in between), rugby now boasts more than eight thousand players nationwide, with more than a quarter of them at the high school level. And the numbers continue to grow each year.

Because rugby requires the endurance and running exertion of soccer, players do face a risk of tendinitis or bursitis of the hips and knees. If pain does develop, ice and rest, combined with gentle stretching exercises, can help alleviate the pain and should be undertaken at the first warning signs of achiness or soreness to avoid more serious wear to the joints.

Far more concerning from a health care provider's perspective are the traumatic and catastrophic injuries that can result from rugby's football-like tackles, called "scrums." And since rugby requires far less protective gear than football, the chance for injury is much higher. In fact, mouth guards are generally the only equipment worn. A mouth guard that fits correctly and provides adequate protection to the entire mouth is therefore especially important.

Head and face injuries are probably the most troubling, especially since helmets are not worn in rugby. Collisions with other players and with the ground can cause everything from a broken nose and black eyes to concussions and fractured skulls. If a player does sustain head trauma— even something seemingly minor—he or she should be evaluated by a medical professional before returning to the game. Remember that a player need not lose consciousness for a concussion to have occurred. You can read about concussions in more detail in chapter 31, but bear in mind that any indication of confusion, dizziness, or blurred vision is a warning sign of a concussion. He should not be permitted to reenter the game. This will heighten his risk of sustaining another injury, and repeated concussions can threaten the long-term health of an athlete's brain. Also, if there is any visible bruising or bleeding on the face or scalp, the player should not return to the field until he has been examined. Even if a player insists that he is fine and a trainer or physician clears him for play, it is advisable that the injury be iced and the player rested for at least ten to fifteen minutes. If a more serious injury to the head or neck is suspected, clear the field and do not allow anyone to move the injured player until a medical team arrives. Even slight movement of the body following a spinal cord injury can result in serious damage, unless conducted by professionals with the correct bracing and stabilization equipment.

The knees are also at risk due to the cutting nature of the sport. When players change direction quickly while trying to evade a defender or block an opponent, the momentum of the body, as well as the possible impact of a colliding player, can cause the knee to twist or torque at an unnatural angle, resulting in a torn anterior cruciate ligament. If an ACL tear occurs, the player usually will not be able to support his weight on the leg, nor should he be encouraged to do so. The player should be carried from the field and examined immediately by a medical professional to determine the extent of the injury. Surgery will be necessary to repair the ligament if it has indeed torn; recovery and rehabilitation from the procedure take around six to twelve months. Although it is impossible to eliminate the risk of ACL tears, athletes are well served to undertake conditioning exercises of the quadriceps muscles and flexibility workouts focused on the knees before the season begins. Developed musculature can help create a natural brace for the joint. Athletes should always remember to build strength gradually to avoid overuse injury or muscle strain.

Shoulder injuries can happen in a variety of ways, including contact with the ground, a rough tackle, or even particularly aggressive rucking (where a player is flanked tightly by two or more opposing players). The joint may become dislocated or sprained due to any kind of rough impact; if the player does not have a full range of motion, or if swelling and bruising are visible immediately following impact, this kind of injury is likely. Because the shoulder is an especially difficult joint to immobilize properly for the sake of rest and recovery, the team's trainer should inspect the joint and bind it appropriately. If the joint seems to be dislocated, only a qualified medical professional should attempt to put the bone back into place. It is generally accepted that the certified athletic trainer is perfectly capable of repositioning, or reducing, a dislocated shoulder on the field. However, afterward, a medical doctor should examine the shoulder and order an X-ray.

Broken collarbones can also result from hard falls. If a player seems slump shouldered after a hit and complains of severe pain, he or she may require an X-ray to determine if the clavicle has been fractured and to what degree. While the bone can often be reset manually, surgery is sometimes required in more severe cases.

Admittedly, there is very little I can recommend in terms of injury prevention for rugby players, simply because of the rough nature and minimal protective gear of the sport. However, I can say that if an athlete dedicates an equal amount of time to improving his flexibility as he or she does to endurance and strength training, the joints stand a much better chance of rebounding from stress or injury. By focusing on all the major joints—neck, shoulders, elbows, wrists, hips, knees, and ankles—a player can help to keep them loose and elastic, making them far more durable. Strength training, especially in the legs and the core, also helps the body endure more impact, and rolling balance boards can be a big help with maintaining footing and keeping the body upright despite shifting weight.

All told, the best advice that I can offer to aspiring rugby players and their parents is as follows:

- Educate yourself on the rules of the game and any league-specific rules. These will clarify what types of hits and tackles are legal, and should help establish boundaries regarding just how rough the game can get.
- Be sure to undertake thorough preseason conditioning that focuses equally on endurance, strength, and flexibility.
- Always wear a properly fitting mouth guard.
- Always use proper technique and follow all league rules in both practice and games, especially in higher-risk situations such as tackling, scrumming, and rucking.
- Do not attempt to play in a league above your ability or comfort level.
- Make sure that the team has a qualified medical professional present at all matches and a fully stocked first aid kit.

Although rugby is certainly a rough sport, the players are a dedicated lot, and the culture of camaraderie and postgame celebration with the opposing team teaches players valuable lessons in sportsmanship. Some parents may not be happy about their sons or daughters embracing the sport, but the huge grins after a safe, hard-played match are likely to win over even the toughest critic.

Chapter 22

Running

Running is so foundational to so many sports that its significance can be considered in a number of different ways. It works in conjunction with an athlete's primary sport (consider soccer or lacrosse, for example), as well as on its own for track-and-field and cross-country athletes. It is important for recreational joggers who run to clear their minds, blow off steam, or just to keep active, but it is also essential as a cardio workout for athletes who wish to stay in shape during the off-season or as part of a conditioning warm-up.

In fact, it's funny to look at how significant running is in so many activities and then to consider that jogging was considered something of a cultural phenomenon in the 1970s, during what the media dubbed the "running boom." Running has always been recognized as a sport, of course, but thanks to figures such as Frank Shorter, who won the marathon at the 1972 Olympics—the first time an American had done so since 1908—it began to grow in popularity. Shorter's victory was quickly followed by the incredible record-breaking feats of athletes such as college phenom Steve Prefontaine. Soon people from all walks of life (please excuse the pun) were running for fitness and for fun. Running clubs sprang up to make jogging a social event. Celebrities and political figures were also spotted picking up the trend. As Title IX opened up more opportunities for female athletes, women's track and field expanded greatly in the United States until women's track teams equaled the size of men's teams at many high schools and colleges. Because of the relatively minimal amount of equipment needed for a track team to operate, many middle schools and junior highs also fielded track teams, which enabled many interested young people to get involved in organized sports at an earlier age.

It is important to remember, however, that the types of running vary greatly. For example, sprinters, whose specialty is short and intense bursts of speed for short distances, have different training goals and techniques than cross-country runners, whose races cover several (or several dozen) miles. However, the health challenges for all runners are surprisingly consistent, so this chapter will examine some of the important guidelines for safety and the most common injuries endured by runners of all types.

The first thing parents should do is talk to their child about his or her running goals. Is your youngster hoping to try out for the track team? Planning to condition for another sport? Or just looking to stay fit? Maybe the child wants to train for a local 5K race or a run to benefit a charity. Sometimes they are eager to have a parent join them in the activity as a way of spending time together. Make sure that there is clear communication about why running is important to the child, and then discuss the best way to set safe and achievable goals.

Once the training begins, parents should be on the lookout for any changes in their child's normal gait. If they notice a limp or stiffness, they should ask the child about any pain or discomfort while running. Because it is not a contact sport, many runners forget that they are just as vulnerable to injuries as football players. Shin splints, for example, are a very common runner's ailment that can arise when running on hard surfaces such as concrete or asphalt. If the athlete is running on roads rather than on a rubberized track, he or she may begin to feel a sharp pain in the lower leg with each strike of the foot; eventually the pain can become consistent. The challenge, however, is that shin splints are not really a condition on their own as much as a symptom of other conditions, such as overuse of the surrounding muscles or stress fractures in the bone. Icing and anti-inflammatories can help, but rest from running is really the most important part of allowing the pain to ease. Cycling or swimming are good cross-training alternatives for reducing impact on the legs and staying in shape while waiting for the pain to subside. Arch supports or custom orthotics can help prevent shin splints, as can wearing a neoprene sleeve to keep the leg supported and warm. If the pain persists, consult with your physician to rule out stress fractures or compartment syndrome.

Runners are vulnerable to hip and pelvis pain, hurdlers especially. Muscle pulls in the groin can result from an improper warm-up or underdeveloped flexibility. Basic stretches for the pelvis, hips, and hamstrings can greatly reduce the chances of injury. For instance, two beneficial exercises are "butterfly" sits, in which the soles of the feet are placed together and drawn toward the body at a 90-degree angle from the back, and touching your toes while standing and then while sitting. However, training for any of the leaping events in track and field should be conducted only under the supervision of a qualified coach to ensure that the best techniques for preparing muscles and joints are followed.

Growth plate stress injuries can affect the hip and pelvis region, as well as the leg and the wrist. During adolescence and puberty, the body's longer bones have cartilaginous tissue between the widened shaft of the bone and the end of the bone. This cartilage allows it to expand and lengthen—in other words, growth plates allow the body to grow. Bones do not grow from the center out, but from each end, gradually lengthening and thickening as the new material ossifies, or hardens into bone. Meanwhile, the cartilaginous tissue remains at each extremity of the bone. Upon reaching the midteens (for girls) and the upper teens (for boys), the cartilage is replaced fully by solid bone when the growing stops. During a youngster's growth process, the ligaments that connect bones to other bones may be stronger than the actual bone itself. When the growth plate areas of the bone are damaged, however, the ossification may occur sooner and stunt growth. Although this type of injury can happen in response to any traumatic injury, it is often tied to falls sustained in running sports. In fact, some studies indicate that up to 30 percent of fractures suffered by children occur in a growth plate region, and up to 10 percent of those injuries could cause problems with the growth plate later on.

If a child suffers from a decreased range of motion or persistent pain that does not respond to treatment, parents should consult a physician to determine if a growth plate has been damaged. This condition can be difficult for a team trainer to diagnose, and (admittedly) is not usually the first thing to which a concerned parent's mind should jump. Wait no longer than five to seven days if the pain seems severe and the injury shows no sign of healing.

Another common issue for runners is tendinitis in the knee or ankle. Achilles tendinitis occurs when the tendons in the heel are stretched and manipulated beyond their normal capacity. Active adolescents are especially vulnerable to this condition, as their bodies are growing at a rapid rate, which puts additional stress upon the tendon. Since tendon rupture can occur if it continues to be pushed, the safest treatment is to apply ice and rest the joint. Do not completely immobilize it. Instead, try no-impact exercises to strengthen the joint and increase flexibility, such as sitting with the foot elevated and tracing in the air each letter of the alphabet or the numbers one through thirty. This moves the joint in different directions but does not add to the irritation by repeatedly striking it against the ground. Once the pain has subsided, this exercise can be done with very light ankle weights to continue building muscle strength as a kind of natural brace. A so-called tight Achilles tendon, a result of overuse, can lead to all kinds of lower extremity problems, so heel cord stretches should be routine in all running sports. The simplest stretch involves leaning against a wall in a forward lunge position. Keeping your back leg straight and heel on the floor, turn your rear foot slightly inward. Lean forward until you feel a mild stretch in back of the ankle, and count to ten. Repeat the stretch with the other leg.

For tendinitis in the knee (patellar tendinitis), the pain tends to progress in stages. At first, it is triggered only following activity, but as the condition worsens, it will show up during running and impede movement. If patellar tendinitis is left untreated, the tendon may tear fully, requiring surgery. Rest, ice, and anti-inflammatories are therefore very important at the earliest stages to prevent the advancement of the condition.

Runners, regardless of the distance or event, are also prone to foot problems such as ankle or toe sprains and plantar fasciitis. In the case of a sprain, the joint will swell and bruise immediately following trauma; it will need to be rested, iced, and given ongoing compression through a brace or wrap. If the swelling and pain do not subside after a few weeks, further medical intervention may be necessary. Plantar fasciitis, which is pain in the bottom of the foot, comes about when the connective tissue of the sole becomes inflamed. It can be triggered by activities such as running, as well as simply by carrying excess body weight. In runners, plantar fasciitis can contribute to knee and foot pain, so it should be treated promptly. If the affected individual is overweight, losing even ten pounds can mitigate the condition noticeably and possibly eliminate it all together. If the athlete is already at a healthy weight, however, a combination of rest, heat, ice, and stretching can improve the situation. Therapeutic massage can also alleviate the pain, as can orthotics and specially designed running shoes. In more severe cases, injections of corticosteroids can bring down the inflammation. Surgery can be helpful in the most extreme situations, but it is certainly not recommended as the first line of treatment.

Blisters can result from improperly fitting shoes or excessive sweating. Always make sure that shoes and socks fit snuggly without wrinkling or gaping at the toes. Also, be sure to purchase the proper type of shoe for your type of running. A regular tennis shoe is fine for casual activity, but if a young person is looking to pursue running seriously, consider investing in shoes and socks specially designed for distance running or sprinting. Even something as seemingly minor as a blister on the heel can greatly impact the efficacy of a workout. A small shake of powder in the shoe or directly on the foot can help protect from moisture, which tends to exacerbate blisters. (Applied to the chest or inner legs, powder can also help prevent heat rash. A small bottle of talcum or cornstarch powder should be a staple in every runner's training bag.)

Leg cramps can debilitate sprinters and distance runners. The muscle spasms are often triggered by a lack of the mineral potassium, which can be combated effectively by eating a banana. Dehydration can also contribute to muscle cramps, so runners should stay adequately hydrated by drinking a minimum of sixteen ounces of water within an hour before working out, and by eating increased helpings of fresh fruits and vegetables during a training regimen. Chest cramps, often described as a "stitch in the side," are the result of shallow breathing. Slowing down to take several deep breaths that expand the lungs can help to alleviate this pain as well as regulate breathing to a more normal state. If this stitch doesn't go away, it can be helpful for the runner to place her hands over her head; this posture naturally opens up the chest and lungs and allows for deeper breathing to occur naturally.

Climate absolutely needs to be taken into account whenever a young athlete is looking to run. As simple as it may sound, applying sunscreen before a run—even on overcast or cool days—can help protect exposed skin from sun damage, including blisters, which can affect both short- and long-term health. Children and teens have a lower tolerance for extreme heat and cold than adults do, so parents should be aware of the forecast and suggest alternate workout times or plans if the temperature is expected to reach 85 degrees or higher, or 45 degrees or lower.

No matter what the temperature is, however, runners should always begin hydrating well before training. Ideally, they should begin to increase their water intake twenty-four hours prior to working out and sustain that level for the duration of the run and in the hours afterward. A water bottle should be carried during long runs—there are many with built-in handles for easy gripping. If the runner is practicing sprints, a water fountain or cooler should be located nearby to provide easy access to liquids. If an athlete is a regular runner, he or she may want to consider carrying a water bottle at all times in order to keep fluid levels high. This not only helps the runner be better prepared for the workout but also helps to increase performance, reduce cramping, and improve recovery.

If a runner does show signs of heat-related illness, swift action must be taken. Once the body reaches a rectal temperature of 104 degrees Fahrenheit, medical personnel have roughly ten minutes to lower the temperature; if the body reaches 105, heatstroke will set in, and vital organs will begin to fail. Therefore, ice baths should be available at longer events, such as 10Ks and marathons, as there is probably not enough time to get the runner to a hospital.

Finally, runners should consider some basic safety precautions before going out jogging. Always make sure that there is clear communication about the proposed route and duration of a run. Carrying a cell phone in a bag or running pack may seem cumbersome, but phones are small enough these days that it should be a nonnegotiable point in the case of injury, danger, losing one's way, or simply an unforeseen delay. Running with a buddy is also advisable. Reflective gear and light-colored clothing are important safety precautions, of course, but runners should also consider going without headphones or keeping the volume very low so that external noises such as traffic can still be detected easily. When possible, runners should always use sidewalks rather than the road. (In some states, it is illegal to run in the road if there is an adjacent sidewalk.) And always run *against* the flow of traffic. This allows both the runner and drivers to see each other better.

Whether running for its own sake or to bolster performance in another sport, running is great activity that can lay the foundation for a lifetime of physical fitness if carried out safely and with a proper understanding of how to prevent injuries early on.

Chapter 23
Skiing and Snowboarding

As I write this, we are still reminded of the tragic death of Canadian freestyle skier Sarah Burke in January 2012, reviving the discussion that seems to arise every time another high-profile figure endures a traumatic head injury on the slopes: What can be done to make skiing and snowboarding safer? The 2009 death of actress Natasha Richardson prompted the question, as did the 1997 and 1998 deaths (only a week apart) of Michael Kennedy, son of Robert F. Kennedy, and Congressman Sonny Bono. Unlike Burke, the three others were just recreational skiers, not engaging in serious training or spending the majority of their time on the mountain. Also, unlike Burke, neither Richardson, Kennedy, nor Bono was wearing a helmet. As Burke's terrible ordeal shows, helmets cannot completely eliminate the risk of injury; however, the US Consumer Product Safety Commission states that helmets could prevent approximately 44 percent of head injuries among all skiers and snowboarders, and up to 53 percent of head injuries for children fifteen and under. Other groups put the estimates as high as 60 percent. When we speak of helmets, it is important to note that there is a difference between wearing a helmet only for style versus wearing a certified helmet for skull protection.

Injuries to the head, neck, or spine—clearly the most serious risks on the slopes or cross-country skiing tracks—account for close to 20 percent of all injuries sustained by skiers and snowboarders ages fifteen and under. Boys are more than twice as likely to suffer injury as girls. Young skiers should always wear protective gear, starting with a snug helmet that is neither too loose nor too tight. Sizes tend to vary among brands, so talk with an associate at the store and consult the brand's sizing charts to determine the best fit. If you don't wish to invest in a helmet because the child is not a regular skier or the family is just preparing to go on a onetime ski vacation, call ahead to ensure that the resort includes helmets as an option in rental packages. Prices are usually below $10 a day and well worth the investment.

In addition to providing UV protection, goggles can shield the eyes from sharp objects, such as tree branches or rocks, if the child slides off the groomed portion of the slope. Although it may seem counterintuitive, the sun can actually pose quite a risk to skiers and snowboarders. Even though the temperatures may be cold, the reflection of the sun on the white snow can magnify its intensity, causing damage to unprotected eyes and burning exposed skin. Always make sure to apply sunscreen with a minimum SPF of 30 to the face before hitting the slopes and to reapply it periodically throughout the day. Be sure to remain hydrated as well. Athletes may not sense it, but they can still sweat just as much in the cold. Perspiration evaporates quickly in the wind, leaving the body dehydrated. Pause for a short break to warm up and rehydrate every two hours to stay on top of fluid levels.

One of the most clichéd images associated with snow sports is the person sitting in the lodge with his or her leg in a cast—and for good reason. While sprains and bruises are common for downhill and cross-country skiers and snowboarders alike, they can usually be treated by resting the limb or bracing the joint until the pain subsides. However, athletes should be aware of any warning signs that there may be a more serious injury. If a sprain is accompanied by bruising over the bone, or if the tissue surrounding a bruise becomes hard, consult a physician and do not return to the slopes or trails until cleared to do so.

More serious injuries, such as fractures, can result from any number of factors, including falls or striking stationary objects, and can result in growth plate injuries. (See chapter 22 for a more detailed discussion.) Although accidents can occur anywhere, the danger factor rises significantly when the skier or snowboarder leaves marked trails or skies out of bounds. Heavier, ungroomed snow is much more difficult to maneuver in smoothly and can also disguise rocks and small tree branches. Additionally, closed trails or areas that are otherwise cordoned off are not patrolled as frequently as the rest of the slopes; therefore, if a fall should occur, help is much farther away. Parents should make it very clear to their children that leaving marked trails is dangerous and that all signs and warnings around the mountain are posted for their protection.

Skiers are at a higher risk for ACL tears than snowboarders. Because both legs are bound to the same surface in snowboarding, the chances of torquing one joint away from the rest of the body is lower. For skiers, who have two separate devices to manage, the odds are much higher. One of the most important tools in protecting the knees is breakaway binding on the skis. The device that keeps the boot locked into the ski will release upon impact. It is essential that skiers have their bindings checked by an expert before the start of the season, and periodically throughout. A binding that is too loose can cause the boot to detach from the ski, causing the athlete to lose his or her balance and fall; an overly tight binding can cause the leg to twist with the ski in a fall, damaging one or both knees. If a skier feels a sharp, piercing sensation or a *pop* in his or her knee during a fall, there may be a fractured bone or torn ligament; it is important to remain still and not try to get back up. The skier's companions should alert the ski patrol or the employees at the ski lift, who can call for help.

While skiers run a higher risk of leg injuries, snowboarders run a higher risk of shoulder, hand, and wrist injuries. Skiers have poles to help them stay upright, but snowboarders have only their arms for trying to maintain their balance. Wrist sprains, fractures, and dislocated shoulders can be incredibly painful and debilitating. Although it is impossible to avoid all falls, preparing for the season by practicing on a rolling balance board can be an excellent way to help the body adapt to shifting weight and momentum, keep the knees loose and flexible, and develop arm balance.

If injury on the slopes does occur, immobilize the joint and seek medical attention if there is visible bruising or if the elbow or shoulder exhibits a limited range of motion. If a dislocation is suspected, immobilize the joint until a diagnosis can be made by a qualified professional; only a certified medical professional should attempt to manipulate the joint back into place. It is best to treat dislocations right away on the slopes.

Both downhill and cross-country skiers are not immune to upper extremity injuries, and the most common is damage to the thumb. If the hand gets tangled in the handle of the pole during a fall, the thumb can either jam into the handle or be twisted at an unnatural angle, causing stress or even a tear to the ligament. If the thumb is bruised, swollen, painful in the joint, and tender to the touch (especially on the inside, near the pointer finger), or if the skier is unable to grip the pole after a fall, there may be damage to the finger. A physician should be consulted for a proper diagnosis to make sure that there is no broken bone in the hand or wrist causing or compounding the pain. If ligament damage is identified as the culprit, surgical intervention may be necessary to correct the problem and restore proper movement and gripping ability to the hand.

Finally, skiers and snowboarders should pay attention to the weather, heeding warnings of any approaching storms, high winds, or dangerously cold temperatures. It goes without saying that proper attire should be worn at all times; however, the bodies of children and teens are generally not as able to withstand extremes of temperature as are adult bodies. Young skiers and snowboarders should take breaks every two hours to sit inside a heated ski lodge and warm up, even if just for fifteen minutes, before returning to the slopes or tracks. These breaks will help the body maintain a healthy temperature, as well as give athletes a chance to rehydrate and rest. Skiers and snowboarders should also make sure to select boots with enough room for them to wiggle their toes should they start to feel numb. Simply moving the toes for forty-five seconds to a minute can improve blood flow and warm the tissue, although the athlete should seek warmth immediately and remain indoors if frostbite is a concern. Until the skin can maintain warmth, the affected individual should not go back outside; repeated warming and cooling of the extremities can increase the damage of frostbite. Pay attention to the color of the fingers, toes, or any other skin that has been exposed to freezing temperatures. If it appears white or ashy (depending on the person's natural skin tone), gradually warm the area with water that is at a temperature comfortable to unaffected body parts; if water is not available, breathe into your cupped hands and hold them against the affected area until the skin turns pink or red. *Do not apply direct heat* such as heating pads, heat packs, or even very hot water. This can cause further tissue damage. Frostbite is a very serious medical condition that can result in the loss of extremities if untreated. Seek out medical attention immediately.

Similarly, hypothermia occurs when the body's temperature drops below 95 degrees. The individual may become confused and sleepy and begin breathing shallowly. If this is the case, transfer the person indoors at once and remove any wet clothing. Wrap the individual in blankets to begin a steady but gradual warming process. Focusing on the chest and trunk of the body, apply warming packs or hot water bottles only if they are covered in cloth and not in direct contact with the skin; starting at the extremities or applying too much direct heat at once can cause the body to go into shock. Do not immerse the affected individual in warm water, as this can disrupt the heartbeat. Make sure that the head is covered to conserve more heat. If the individual is able to swallow, administer warm (but not hot) nonalcoholic and decaffeinated beverages. Contact emergency medical professionals if the affected individual does not seem to respond to the warming efforts or if he or she loses consciousness.

Skiing and snowboarding are dynamic, exciting sports that combine speed, skill, and a rush of adrenaline—everything that adventurous young people seem to love. The good news is that the past decade has seen a tremendous increase in the use of safety equipment by participants; the bad news is that there is still a long way to go. Any young person interested in starting in snow sports should take lessons before attempting to hit the slopes independently. Classes are available for all age groups and will teach the fundamentals of movement, stopping, and correct technique, as well as matching aspiring athletes with correctly fitting equipment. With a little preparation and common sense about safety, skiing and snowboarding can be wonderful ways to stay active in the winter and grow as an athlete.

Chapter 24
Soccer

Soccer—also called association football, or just football in other countries—has existed in its modern form only since 1863 but has become the most popular game in the world, with more than 250 million players in more than two hundred countries spanning the globe. Thanks in large part to its minimal equipment requirements, it is as popular in developing nations as it is in industrialized ones; anyone can play if he has a couple of goal boundaries and something that can roll when kicked, even if it's just a bundle of rags tied into a ball. In the United States, which has traditionally favored other sports, soccer has become one of the fastest-growing sports over the past thirty years, expanding widely in both boys' and girls' leagues. Interestingly, girls' soccer is one of the leading sources of injury in youth sports—a statistic we'd like to see changed.

In fact, parents should also be aware that girls' soccer is second only to football in the number of concussions in youth sports. Concussions are discussed in detail in chapter 31, but parents should be aware that a concussion may still have occurred even if the athlete does not lose consciousness. Therefore, it is extremely important that coaches and parents learn how to recognize the warning signs of a concussion and remove the player from the game until he or she can be evaluated by a medical professional. Any player who seems confused, dizzy, or unfocused after a fall involving the head should get professional attention before returning to play, and be watched closely for any changes in behavior, sleep patterns, or emotional health for several weeks afterward, as these can all be late-onset symptoms of a concussion.

Without question, however, the most common injuries in soccer are sprains and strains in the lower legs. As with any such injury, RICE (rest, ice, compression, elevation) treatment is the first step. Any player nursing a sprained ankle should expect to be off his or her feet for a minimum of a week, possibly longer. If sharp pain persists beyond a week, or if bruising and swelling do not subside, medical intervention may be necessary to rule out a fracture or other serious injury to the joint or bone. A preseason conditioning regimen and thorough leg stretching routine are the best ways to prepare the body for safe play. Gradually adding weight and repetitions to leg presses and calf exercises will strengthen the muscles so that they serve as a natural brace to the joints. Stretching each major muscle group both before and after workouts will help keep the body limber and increase flexibility. These preparations will allow joints to endure stress without damage. Soccer players should also train for endurance, combining cardio with strengthening workouts. Swimming and cycling are good options for soccer players who want to cross-train, as they minimize the amount of stress put on the lower body while steadily increasing the body's ability to remain active for extended periods of time.

Severe bruising is also common in soccer players and often stems from contact between the body and ball or impact with other players. If a bruise (also called a contusion) is exceptionally large, painful, or becomes hard, athletes should consult their team's trainer. Because the accompanying discoloration is the result of broken capillaries leaking blood beneath the surface of the skin, any contusion that seems out of the ordinary should receive medical attention. Most bruises, however, are relatively minor and should show signs of healing within a few days; they are to be an expected part of an active child or teen's life.

More serious injuries common to soccer players include meniscal tears and ACL damage. In fact, ACL injuries have one of the highest incidents in girls' soccer over all other sports. If there is a popping sound in the joint either at the time of the accident or immediately following it, or if there is limited range of motion and swelling accompanied by intense pain, the athlete should be removed from the game immediately and given prompt medical attention. If an ACL tear has occurred, the joint will not bear weight, so the athlete must be carried from the field; he or she should not attempt to walk on the injured joint. An MRI may be required to confirm the diagnosis, at which point surgical repair will be necessary, as the ligament cannot repair itself on its own. While the recovery and rehabilitation period from ACL surgery is approximately six to twelve months, the recovery rate is very high, and athletes can usually plan to rejoin their teams for the next season.

Not all soccer injuries occur in the legs, however; the upper extremities are also at risk. Wrist sprains and fractures, as well as elbow or shoulder dislocations, can occur when a player tries to catch himself or herself when falling or simply from impact with the ground or another player. All types of dislocations are serious. A simple dislocation means that while the bones in the joint have been displaced, there is no serious damage to them. Simple dislocations can usually be manually manipulated back into place by an athletic trainer or doctor, and will require splinting or other means of immobilization for several weeks. Only a physician or other certified medical professional should attempt to realign the joint.

A complex dislocation, on the other hand, is a serious injury to the bones, ligaments, or both. Surgery may be required to repair the damage before the joint can be realigned. A severe dislocation can damage the nerves and blood vessels serving the joint and, in the most extreme cases, lead to limb loss. The circulation should be evaluated by checking the pulse if the arm has been injured and making sure that the hand is the proper color and still warm rather than cool, tingling, or numb, the latter of which may imply damage to the blood vessels. A partial dislocation may not appear to be a problem immediately, as the joint is only slightly out of place and may correct itself without any medical assistance if it is treated with caution and kept from unnecessary activity. However, if pain and bruising around the joint linger for a few weeks, the injury may require medical attention to make sure the ligaments are healing properly.

If a joint suffers trauma that inhibits range of motion or causes it to bend at an unnatural angle, the athlete should be examined by a medical professional. Any dislocation will likely require some degree of rehabilitation or physical therapy to restore full joint movement; athletes eager to rejoin their team will need to be patient while the joint heals fully. Many athletes will wear some type of harness or stabilization device once they return.

Stress fractures, shin splints, and tendinitis in either the knee or the ankle are also common injuries in soccer. Fortunately, proper stretching and conditioning can help alleviate many of the symptoms. Core-strengthening exercises can also help athletes avoid overuse injuries to the lower extremities by counteracting poor posture or sloppy form when fatigue sets in toward the end of a match. Ice and over-the-counter anti-inflammatory medicines can help reduce the pain; however, the best treatment is rest.

Parents should be aware that taking a break from the sport makes a significant difference in how a young athlete's body holds up under the stress of competition. With the explosive growth of indoor and year-round soccer teams over the past two decades, aspiring players can now play twelve months a year—but this is not a healthy option. Pursuing alternative sports or activities will help them not only stay in shape but also work different muscles, develop different skills, and avoid burnout or overuse in the off-season. The hairline cracks, or stress fractures, that develop in a bone as a result of overuse significantly weaken the bone. This puts the athlete at a higher risk for an acute fracture, which will be far more painful and potentially hazardous to his or her future. By reducing activity and giving the body sufficient time to rest and recover, an athlete can actually be making a greater investment in his or her talent than continually pushing through the pain.

Elite training academies and travel teams have also become a staple of the sport, as budding athletes look to gain an advantage over competitors. These programs can cost tens of thousands of dollars each year to attend, and require a tremendous amount of time as well. Some academies function like boarding schools, where students live in dorms and attend a shortened academic school day before drilling and practicing in the afternoon. These may range from summer- or semester-long programs to year-round, full-time schools. Selective travel teams also require extensive travel, sometimes on weekends and sometimes actually during the school week as well. Parents and athletes should give serious consideration to the level of commitment they are willing to give to the sport, all other costs aside. It is also important for mothers and fathers to remember that players who are feeling burned out on the game often feel too guilty to speak up because of the money and time their parents have already invested. If a once-enthusiastic child begins to find excuses to miss practice or workouts, talk to him or her about why. It could be that he or she is stressed from school or perhaps having a personality clash with another player on the team; on the other hand, it could just be that the child is feeling worn out and wants to take a break from the sport but does not wish to disappoint anyone. Make sure that there is an open line of communication so that young athletes can ask for a break from training if they begin to feel overwhelmed or disheartened by their pursuit of soccer.

Chapter 25
Softball

Softball is one of the most popular sports among children, teens, and adults alike. Between work leagues, community teams, and church groups, it seems like everyone belongs to a softball team these days—and I couldn't be more delighted! What a wonderful way for adults to stay active, blow off some steam, and build relationships with coworkers and friends.

Though adult leagues are often coed, youth softball is almost exclusively a girls' sport—and those young ladies can look up to some great heroines. In fact, at the time this book went to press, Team USA had won three consecutive gold medals in the Olympic Games in 1996, 2000, and 2004, and a silver in 2008 before softball was eliminated as an Olympic sport. Team USA has finished either first or second in the World Cup of Softball every year it's been played since the inaugural event in 2005. I want to make a few recommendations for keeping the game and its players as safe as possible to ensure that this streak of excellence continues.

The first thing to remember is that there is a big difference between fast-pitch and slow-pitch softball. Slow-pitch is usually reserved for girls in elementary school and middle school; in fact, in some leagues, any pitch judged to be too fast is called a ball. I heartily approve the rule both for the safety of the batter, who, at eight or nine years old is unlikely to have the eye-hand coordination to make contact with a fastball, as well as for the pitcher, who is likely to suffer elbow and shoulder injuries if she is required to throw that hard at such an early age. In addition, slow-pitch leagues allow younger girls a chance to learn the fundamentals of the game. I urge all parents to keep their children in slow-pitch leagues until at least age eleven or twelve. It will not only help protect their bodies and thus prolong their careers but can also take some of the fiercely competitive edge off the game and keep it more fun, which helps prevent burnout.

Fast-pitch is the standard version of the game for high school, college, and professional leagues, and it is here that the most injuries take place. One of the biggest challenges in softball is the sport's rigorous schedule. Some athletes may play up to six games in one weekend. Unfortunately, softball lags behind all other youth sports in injury rate recognition and preventative safety rules. There have been very few rules regulating softball at any level and, as a result, softball injuries in young athletes are on the rise and are nearly as prevalent as baseball injuries.

Thankfully, the Little League International Association has stepped up to change this by setting softball pitch-count guidelines similar to those in baseball. Obviously, the focus on pitchers' health is the main concern, as their bodies incur unique stresses. Catchers and infielders are also at risk; however, most softball teams usually rely on one or two girls to pitch all the innings of all the games in a weekend tournament. To protect these young women, Little League International now recommends the following guidelines:

- The maximum pitch count for eight- to ten-year-olds is 50 or a combined two-day total of 80. Pitchers should not throw more than two games in a row.
- For ages ten to twelve, pitches per game are limited to 65 or a combined two-day total of 95. Again, pitchers should not throw more than two games in a row.

- For ages thirteen to fourteen, pitches per game are limited to 80, or a combined two-day total of 115. Pitches per day for days one and two are 115; pitches for day three are 80.
- For ages fifteen and over, pitches per game are limited to 100, or a combined two-day total of 140; pitches for day three are 100.

Pitchers' injuries certainly differ from those of other positions because pitchers use a powerful dynamic windmill motion that places a unique demand on the back, neck, shoulder, elbow, forearm, and wrist. It is not uncommon for young windmill pitchers to have significant shoulder instability patterns, with tears to the labrum and the rotator cuff. Tommy John ligament (ulnar collateral ligament) injuries are also common. Previously, it was thought that pitching underhanded did not damage the throwing arm; not only is this untrue, but I must remind all parents and young softball pitchers that throwing with the modern windmill pitching technique is *not* the same as throwing underhanded. If anyone tries to argue with you on this point, you can tell them I say that's pure malarkey. Softball-related overuse injuries of the shoulder and elbow that require surgical intervention are quite common today and are on the rise, whereas I almost never saw such cases when I first started in sports medicine.

For pitchers, the most common overuse injury is shoulder tendinitis—that is, inflammation of the tendons that make up the rotator cuff. Any athlete complaining of pain in her shoulder should be taken out of the rotation immediately and allowed to rest until the pain has subsided. Ice and anti-inflammatories can reduce swelling, but she should not return to the game until her shoulder feels better without medication or ice and after she has regained her shoulder dynamic stability and neuromuscular control through rehabilitation. By allowing her body to rest at the first sign of strain, she can help protect the long-term stability and health of her joint. Preseason conditioning that focuses on shoulder strength and muscular development is also recommended to prepare the joint. However, it is essential to remember that all weight training should progress gradually; otherwise you run the risk of an overuse injury before the season even begins.

Tendinitis in the forearm and wrist are also risks for pitchers, as are back and neck pain. At the first sign of tenderness in the arm or soreness along the spine, the athlete should be removed from play and allowed to rest. Keep in mind that rest means no live pitches, including batting practice. If a pitcher is feeling well enough to throw on two consecutive days, she may need to loosen up with a flexibility routine on the second rest day before hitting and fielding drills.

As in baseball, catchers have their own unique set of concerns. As the workhorses of the team, these athletes throw almost as much as pitchers, and must also leap up out of their crouch to corral foul pop-ups and tag runners out at home. As a result, their shoulders should be iced and rested regularly to avoid overuse. Catchers' knees and backs also endure a lot of stress from the crouching position. Proper safety gear can help provide some cushioning and protection, but preseason conditioning of the core muscles may be a catcher's best defense against muscle strains and fatigue. By gradually building up the muscles in the abdomen, lower back, and legs, catchers can create a kind of natural brace for their joints as the body stabilizes itself. If a catcher has pain in her knees following practice or a game, she should talk with her coach about modifying her stance; additionally, she should take care to rest her knees before playing again, to ensure that she is not damaging the joint further.

For other position players, shoulder and elbow pain tend to be the most common complaints. Due to physical development and genetics, many young women have a natural laxity of the shoulders and lack of dynamic stabilization. Since some female athletes are reluctant to "bulk up" their shoulder muscles through repetitive weight-lifting regimens, I often recommend that softball players perform throwing exercises to develop the dynamics of their shoulder. This will gradually build strength in the joint and prevent inherent overuse and laxity problems, which are generally the source of labral and rotator cuff injuries. Athletes and parents should talk with the coach about the best and safest techniques for overhand throws.

Many softball injuries are preventable, especially those resulting from overuse. Some guidelines to keep young athletes in the game for life are as follows:

1. Young softball players should warm up properly with stretching, running, and easy, gradual throwing.

2. Coaches should rotate pitchers to other positions. Additionally, the pitcher and catcher should not necessarily switch positions. It is easy to overuse the best athlete on a youth softball team and cause lasting joint damage from overuse in the process.

3. Coaches and parents should concentrate on age-appropriate pitching. The more complicated windmill-type pitches should be left to mature pitchers as they approach their senior year in high school and during their college careers. Teams should also adhere to pitch-count guidelines.

4. Adequate rest periods for pitchers and catchers are essential.

5. Avoid pitching on multiple teams with overlapping seasons. A young softball player should never play on two softball teams at the same time.

6. For pitchers, flexibility needs to be the focus during the season rather than strengthening.

7. Don't allow a pitcher to play with pain, and have her see a trainer, physical therapist, or sports doctor if pain persists for a week.

8. Pitchers should not throw on more than two consecutive days until age thirteen, and then no more than three days in a row.

9. To avoid fatigue and burnout, don't play year-round. Instead, try cross-training with a sport that utilizes different muscle groups, such as soccer or cycling.

10. The emphasis on pitch velocity is a major factor in overuse injuries. The only reason to ever use a radar gun in softball is to check the differences in velocity between a pitcher's fastball and changeup in competition. Radar guns should not be used until the pitcher is a minimum of fifteen years old.

11. Make sure that players feel they can communicate regularly about

how their arms are feeling and that any concerns will be taken seriously by coaches and the team's athletic trainers or other health care professionals.

12. Develop only skills that are age appropriate.

13. Remember that specialization and the word *professionalism* should never be stressed among preteens and teenagers.

14. Emphasize control for accuracy and good mechanics. Poor mechanics is still the number one reason for injury in softball, as well as in other sports that call for overhand throwing or hitting.

15. Speak with a sports medicine professional or athletic trainer if there are any concerns about injuries or prevention strategies.

16. Return to play only when clearance is granted by a health care professional.

I encourage advanced softball pitchers to study the Interval Throwing Program used at the American Sports Medicine and the Andrews Institute and included here. It is a good regimen to follow.

Softball Phase I Interval Throwing Program
(position players)

30' Phase

STEP 1:
        A) Warm-up throwing
        B) 30' (25 throws)
        C) Rest 15 minutes
        D) Warm-up throwing
        E) 30' (25 Throws)

STEP 2:
        A) Warm-up throwing
        B) 30' (25 throws)
        C) Rest 10 minutes

     D) Warm-up throwing
     E) 30' (25 throws)
     F) Rest 10 minutes
     G) Warm-up throwing
     H) 30' (25 throws)

45' Phase

STEP 3:
     A) Warm-up throwing
     B) 45' (25 throws)
     C) Rest 15 minutes
     D) Warm-up throwing
     E) 45' (25 throws)

STEP 4:
     A) Warm-up throwing
     B) 45' (25 throws)
     C) Rest 10 minutes
     D) Warm-up throwing
     E) Rest 10 minutes
     F) Warm-up throwing
     G) 45' (25 throws)

60' Phase

STEP 5:
     A) Warm-up throwing
     B) 60' (25 throws)
     C) Rest 15 minutes
     D) Warm-up throwing
     E) 60' (25 throws)

STEP 6:
     A) Warm-up throwing
     B) 60' (25 throws)
     C) Rest 10 minutes

D) Warm-up throwing

E) 60' (25 throws)

F) Rest 10 minutes

G) Warm-up throwing 60' (25 throws)

90' Phase

STEP 7:

A) Warm-up throwing

B) 90' (25 throws)

C) Rest 15 minutes

D) Warm-up throwing

E) 90' (25 throws)

STEP 8:

A) Warm-up throwing

B) 90' (20 throws)

C) Rest 10 minutes

D) Warm-up throwing

E) 60' (20 throws)

F) Rest 10 minutes

G) Warm-up throwing

H) 45' (20 throws)

I) Rest 10 minutes

J) Warm-up throwing

K) 45' (15 throws)

30 feet = 9.1 meters; 45 feet = 13.7 meters; 60 feet = 18.3 meters;
90 feet = 27.4 meters

Interval Throwing Program—Windmill Softball Pitchers—Phase II

Throwing program to be completed by windmill softball pitchers following
successful completion of Phase I interval throwing program. Perform throwing
from mound every other day, three days per week. Continue all thrower's
resistance exercises, stretching, hitting drills, and other throwing drills in
addition to this off-the-mound throwing program.

STEP 1:

>   Warm-up at 100-foot phase
>   20 windmill at 50% intensity

STEP 2:

>   Warm-up at 100-foot phase
>   30 windmill at 50% intensity

STEP 3:

>   Warm-up at 100-foot phase
>   40 windmill at 50% intensity
>   15 windmill at 75% intensity

STEP 4:

>   Warm-up at 100-foot phase
>   20 windmill at 50% intensity
>   35 windmill at 75% intensity

STEP 5:

>   Warm-up at 100-foot phase
>   50 windmill at 75% intensity
>   15 windmill at 50% intensity

STEP 6:

>   Warm-up at 100-foot phase
>   60 windmill at 75% intensity
>   15 batting practice throws

STEP 7:

>   Warm-up at 100-foot phase
>   40 windmill at 75% intensity
>   10–15 windmill at 90% intensity
>   20 breaking balls at 50% intensity
>   30 batting practice throws

STEP 8:

>   Warm-up at 100-foot phase
>   30 windmill at 75% intensity

10–15 windmill at 90–100%
30 breaking balls at 75% intensity
30 batting practice throws

STEP 9:

Simulated game
Gradually increase number of breaking balls and total numbers of pitches

STEP 10:

Competition
Gradually return to competition
May use pitch count if necessary

The main thing about youth softball is that someone has to take the bull by the horns and recognize that injuries are on the rise. These young women need to be protected for the sake of their long-term health, not just for their team's win-loss record. We must make softball a safer sport for the thousands of young women who love it.

Chapter 26
Swimming

Who can forget the unbelievable excitement of watching Michael Phelps slice through the water, stroke after stroke, at the Beijing Olympics? His incredible eight gold medals at the 2008 Games made him a national icon and doubtlessly inspired scores of children to don swimming caps and goggles and take to the pool in the hopes of replicating a little bit of Phelps's Olympic glory.

Swimming enjoys an incredible amount of variety, with forty different events recognized by the Federation Internationale de Natation (FINA), the international governing body of water sports. Various strokes, distances, relays, and endurance events mean that swimmers can adapt their interests based on personal preference and talent. Water therapy is also growing in popularity as a low-impact way to stay fit or recover from injuries in other sports. However, swimming is also a sport that requires a great deal of time and dedication on the part of both athletes and parents. Some communities have swim teams at neighborhood or municipal pools, but practice hours are restricted to early mornings and evenings so as not to interfere with pool access for casual swimmers, water aerobics classes, senior citizens doing low-impact workouts, people rehabilitating hips and knees, and recreational swimmers. Many schools have swim teams, but not all have swimming pools; as a result, swimmers must be transported to and from practice facilities. Some teams practice twice a day to make up for their limited time in the water. Combine this with a full day at school and work, plus homework, household chores, and everything else in everyday life, and the stress can mount very quickly. That's not to mention all-day swim meets on weekends. But for those who love it, there is no better smell than chlorine in the water and no better feeling than a well-executed flip-turn and touching the wall fractions of a second ahead of the swimmer in the next lane.

Swimmers are a dedicated bunch; there is no question about it. But because they tend to be such determined devotees to their sport, it is easy for many young athletes to overtrain in pursuit of their goals. As a result, most swimming injuries stem from overuse. Traumatic injuries can occur, but they are usually secondary dangers, such as diving into shallow water or swimming alone. It goes without saying that swimmers should always heed warning signs about depth and water conditions, and should practice under supervision; even the most experienced swimmers can suddenly develop cramps or accidentally inhale water in such a way that poses a drowning threat.

The most likely danger that young swimmers face, however, is joint damage, with the shoulder bearing the lion's share of the stress. When the tendons in the biceps become inflamed, biceps tendinitis results, which can make any rotation of the arm painful. The condition can result from fatigue, which leads to improper stroke technique, as well as overuse. Similarly, shoulder instability leads to shoulder misalignment, which causes the ball at the upper end of the humerus (the long bone in the upper arm) to slip from the socket joint. Rotator cuff impingement is a painful condition similar to bursitis, in which the bursa sac becomes irritated from repetitive motion or microtrauma. Impingement results from the shoulder blade pressing on the rotator cuff of the shoulder when the arm is raised; the small blood vessels in the muscle swell and fray due to overuse. Gradual conditioning exercises to build up muscle strength in the shoulder joint and the shoulder blade (scapula) will help to combat all of these injuries.

Flexibility is certainly a good thing, and swimmers tend to be very flexible due to the nature of the joint rotation required for the sport. However, joint laxity and muscular imbalance are not uncommon among swimmers. This can lead to joint damage and sprains, as the bones and tissues are easily moved into positions or angles they were not designed to reach. Because the condition is technically an inherited one rather than something an athlete can develop, it is somewhat difficult to speak to. Many swimmers who are already genetically predisposed to flexibility will find that their joints are especially limber because of the full-body movements required by swimming. Since hyperflexibility poses a higher threat of sprains due to the joint "rolling," it is important that swimmers strengthen the muscles surrounding any joint they find to be overly loose. They should still stretch for flexibility but be careful not to overstretch or overrotate the joint while doing so. Strength conditioning workouts using light weight with multiple repetitions will help to bolster the body's natural support and improve joint mobility. Young swimmers should not lift heavy weights or max out. All too often, a football-type workout is prescribed for young adolescent swimmers, which can lead to significant joint injury. Circuit training, a popular approach in which athletes exercise until the point of fatigue, is an injury producer for loose-jointed swimmers. Also, yardage makes a difference. Sprinters who are used to shorter swims should not be subjected to longer distance workouts. Specialists in one stroke should not be required to work out in another stroke except a natural crawl stroke and should especially avoid the butterfly stroke. For example, a sprinter who competes in freestyle should not practice for yardage with a butterfly stroke. Parents should also be aware that children who demonstrate tremendous flexibility or joint laxity tend to be at higher risk for scoliosis, and should make sure that all proper screenings are conducted to detect this potentially life-limiting spinal condition. Elementary and middle schools generally do routine checks during health screenings; pediatricians will also look for it during checkups. With early intervention, scoliosis can usually be treated efficiently; only in rare cases will it prove an uncorrectable problem.

Knee injuries in swimming are so common that one even bears the nickname "breaststrokers' knee." This is an overuse injury wherein the tendons and ligaments in the inner knee become irritated from kick motions. This can lead to subluxation of the kneecap, wherein the kneecap has a tendency to pop out of joint to the outside. It can also occur in the hip tendons. The simplest and best way to combat this condition is to focus on proper technique and to take sufficient rest periods between practice sessions. Dolphin kicks are also important to learn under the guidance of a coach in order to avoid unnecessary strain to the back muscles. More seriously, improperly performed dolphin kicks can lead to spinal disc problems in the lower back, as well as spondylolysis, which is an injury to the vertebrae at the junction of the spine and the pelvis. Core strengthening in the preseason can help prevent these injuries, as can pelvic- and hip-strengthening workouts. The latter can also help prevent knee injuries by strengthening the upper leg and building up the muscle to reinforce the joint.

Aspiring swimmers and parents should also be aware of the differences between the two major seasons recognized in American club swimming: short course and long course. Short-course swimming takes place from late fall to early spring, and competition pools are generally twenty-five meters in length. (Occasionally pools may be twenty-five yards, but the metric measurement tends to be the standard.) This is the format used by the FINA World Swimming Championships. Long-course swimming takes place during the summer months, and the pools are fifty meters, the same length used in Olympic competition. Unless you live in a climate that is warm year-round, short-course swimming takes place in indoor pools or outdoor pools covered with a seasonal "bubble." Ironically, it is often long-course swimmers who have to contend with the cold even though the season is warmer. Early-morning practices outdoors on a spring morning can be extremely chilly. It may be natural that swimmers shiver when first entering the water, and some may even find that their lips turn blue. Movement and activity in the water, uncomfortable as they might be at first, will help to get the blood moving and will help regulate the body's temperature. Parents should keep in mind, however, that children cannot withstand extreme variances in temperatures as readily as adults do. If a child does not show signs of warming up after about ten minutes of continuous exercise in the water, he or she should climb out of the pool and be wrapped in a towel until the shivering stops.

It is also important to speak to athletes who are considering swimming as a means of cross-training or staying in shape during the off-season. I strongly recommend swimming to almost everyone who is looking for a sport that offers a great cardio workout while also keeping the muscles toned and active; the only exception (and it is a large one) is any athlete whose primary sport revolves around throwing, such as baseball or softball. Because the shoulder is so foundational to swimming, anyone seeking to rest his or her arm should look elsewhere. Swimming will only exacerbate any pain, irritation, swelling, or damage already present in the joint. Cross-training is a fantastic, smart pursuit, but athletes do need to be wise in what they choose to pursue in the off-season to keep the body as healthy and injury free as possible. For the rest, however, swimming is an outstanding way to stay in shape and enjoy competition, whether in individual events or as part of a relay. Even those athletes for whom swimming is a secondary sport and are just swimming laps to stay in shape in between seasons, the proper stretches and correct technique will help keep the body in prime condition for a lifetime of fitness.

Chapter 27
Tennis

One of the most popular sports worldwide, and with roots reaching back to the Middle Ages, tennis is a fixture in many communities, schools, and universities. The list of elite competitions—the US Open, the French Open, the Australian Open, and Wimbledon, just to name the four Grand Slam events—are some of the most prestigious tournaments in all of sports and attract millions of television viewers around the world. Singles and doubles; grass, clay, and hard court—the variations within the game require players to adapt their style and strategy while still maintaining the fast-paced, aggressive nature of the game. It is a joy to watch as much as it is to play, and many young athletes are flocking to the sport to get fit and maybe even advance in tournament play, where they can climb in the rankings, gain sponsors, and hone their skills with an eye toward going pro in adult competition.

There is no question that tennis can be a profitable sport for the most elite competitors, and that advancing through the junior levels has proven the surest way of developing skills. However, as athletes are being introduced to tennis at younger and younger ages, they are also running the risk of wearing out their bodies before they have a chance to make it even to the higher levels. Tennis academies, which are essentially boarding schools for promising young tennis players, are becoming increasingly popular among the ambitious. While these schools can certainly provide great instruction and one-on-one coaching, they can also contribute significantly to overuse injuries and burnout. Athletes and parents considering one of these academies should evaluate whether the investment of money (usually in the tens of thousands of dollars) and time (courses typically range from three months to a year) are really worth it for the physical stress it can put on a growing body, not to mention the financial and emotional stress it can place on a family.

If a family does decide that they wish to pursue enrollment in a tennis academy—or even if they just want to hire a private instructor for lessons closer to home—the most important thing to remember is that the risk of overuse injuries correlates directly to the amount of time spent on the court, with two hours being the safety threshold. Two-thirds of all tennis injuries result from overuse, so parents, coaches, and athletes alike need to be aware of the risks associated with overpracticing. Probably no other sport typifies the word *professionalism* at a young age more than tennis.

One of the most common overuse injuries is tennis elbow. It's an injury so closely associated with the sport that it even derives its name from it. When the ball makes contact with the racket or the player swings to hit, these muscles and joints (both in the elbow and the wrist, despite what the name implies) absorb the impact and can become overused and even hyperextended. Proper technique is an obvious fix; however, parents should check the child's equipment to make sure that the racket is of a proper weight and grip size, especially if it's a hand-me-down. Ask your child's coach to inspect the racket to ensure it is appropriate for the child's age, hand, and style of play. Also consider a conditioning workout that gradually builds up the muscles surrounding the wrist and elbow. Light-resistance exercise bands that allow the player to practice wrist flexion can help to strengthen the joints as well as increase flexibility. A simple conditioning workout three to four times a week can help to combat pain and build muscle.

A thorough warm-up routine, like the one pictured in chapter 32, can also help. Consider adding additional stretches that can help limber up the elbow and upper arms, too. For example, raise and bend the right arm so that the elbow is positioned near the top of the head. Then reach over and grasp the right elbow with the left hand and gently push the arm backward. Hold for a count of ten before switching sides. Repeat this three times. Simple techniques like these can help decrease the likelihood of tennis elbow.

Shoulder overuse injuries are usually caused when the tendon or bursa (the fluid-filled sac under the joint) becomes irritated or inflamed. The pain is felt most clearly when serving the ball or hitting an overhead shot. Fatigue in the shoulder can cause the joint to become unstable and create more friction in the socket. If a child complains of shoulder soreness or has any swelling following practice, he or she should take off at least one day to allow the muscles and tendons to rest and repair themselves. If the pain persists or there is a nagging achiness in the joint, it may be necessary to consult a physician to ensure that there is no tear or other undiagnosed problem. Remember that the weight of the racket can cause soreness. Increasing racket weight too quickly can bring about fatigue in the elbow and wrist. Wrist pain can also result from tendinitis and ligament strains, so athletes should be attuned to the state of their entire arm following practice or matches.

Stress fractures are also a very common problem, occurring when athletes train too rapidly. When muscles grow tired, the body naturally adapts its movements so that more stress is put on the bone. If the athlete is not well conditioned, this transition can be too rapid for the bone to absorb the extra demands, and small cracks can result. Most stress fractures among tennis players occur in the leg or foot, and are largely avoidable through proper footwear, strength and endurance training as part of preseason conditioning, and adhering to two-hour practice limits. Footwear is especially important: be sure to look for shoes designed specifically for the flexibility, cushioning, and support tennis necessitates. Shoes should have good traction to help avoid sliding on the court, as well as giving the athlete a good grip for stopping and starting. If a tennis shoe shows the least bit of wear, it should be replaced. Athletes who play primarily on hard-court surfaces are more likely to develop stress fractures, although all tennis players are vulnerable. If the shin or foot hurts after a match or practice session, suspend all activity until the pain resolves itself. Because stress fractures are cumulative (existing cracks may worsen or new ones form as repeated stress to the bone continues), the bone becomes more and more susceptible to serious fractures in which the bone actually snaps or is dislodged from its natural position. A few days of rest at the first sign of pain can make a huge difference in terms of protecting the bone for the long term.

Beyond the more serious conditions, tennis players are vulnerable to more mundane but no less frustrating injuries such as muscle strain. Because these often result from quick or sharp movements such as those that are often necessary in tennis, a low-intensity cardio warm-up followed by thorough stretching (no less than five minutes) can go a long way toward preparing the body for play. Do pay attention to healthy stretching techniques for the entire body. Focus on the joints and muscles that get the heaviest use during tennis, but also make sure that every major muscle group is sufficiently limber. The muscle or joint should never be worked into a position that cannot be held for less than approximately thirty seconds. Never bounce when stretching, either, as this can cause extra stress or tears in the muscle as it is pushed past its normal capacity for movement. Tennis players will benefit from movement stretches, such as large, circular movements with the arms and swinging the leg forward and backward to warm up the hips and knees.

Heat can also be a risk factor. A tennis court is generally about 15 degrees warmer than the air temperature, which means that radiating heat can cause players to become fatigued or dehydrated even faster. Make sure that youngsters drink plenty of water before, during, and after any practice or match, and be sure to take precautions against the sun as well. If an athlete becomes light-headed or dizzy, cease play immediately, move to an air-conditioned or shaded area, and make sure that he or she continues to consume fluids. Do not let the affected individual return to the court until he or she feels strong and stable enough to continue. Remember that children's bodies are less able to handle extreme temperatures than are adults' bodies; do not assume that just because you can stand the heat, your child will be fine as well. It may also be helpful for athletes to wear two pairs of socks to prevent blisters from a court that has absorbed too much heat from the sun. Doubled socks can prevent soreness in the shins due to overheating as well. Always wear sunscreen (at minimum with a sun protection factor of 15, although SPF 30 is better) and avoid sunburn and long-term sun damage with brands that are waterproof or sweatproof.

Finally, parents should stay closely attuned to their child's attitude toward tennis. Because of the amount of time required to train and develop one's game, the risk for burnout is high. If a child who was once enthusiastic about practice is now finding excuses to not go, it may be worth considering a little time off. Sometimes a few weeks or a month away will allow the athlete a chance to miss the sport and return to it with a renewed sense of excitement. Short hiatuses are especially important for those athletes who live in places where tennis can be played year-round, thanks to climate or indoor practice facilities. Allowing the child a chance to explore other sports can help develop muscles through cross-training, or simply letting them rest from sports altogether can help the body have a chance to recover and repair itself in anticipation of the next season.

One of the most distressing anecdotes in my many years of sports medicine occurred with the parents of a young tennis player. I had a phone call one day—completely out of the blue—from parents wanting to know what sports agents I would recommend for their son. As the conversation went on, I learned that the athlete was being shipped off to a tennis "factory" to live and was set to sign an endorsement contract with a major commercial athletic company; thus the need for a sports agent. Finally, it occurred to me to ask how old the tennis player was—and the parents told me *six*!

Physical fitness is a wonderful lifelong habit, but children who are immersed in it too intensely too early can find themselves nursing worn-out shoulders and damaged elbows long before their time. Any young tennis players with aspirations of going pro should take their health as seriously as they take their goals and make safety a regular part of their training regimen.

Chapter 28
Volleyball

Born just four years and ten miles away from basketball, volleyball was first called Mintonette when it was created in Springfield, Massachusetts, in 1895. While it was at first conceived as a way for older adults to enjoy physical activity in the winter without as much player-to-player contact, volleyball is now a sport that many associate with young, fit, tan beachgoers. That's not without good cause, of course: Volleyball is now played as a team sport on the court or as two-against-two in the sand, with both versions of the sport now officially part of Olympic competition. Most youth programs are six-person teams on a wooden court; also, the vast majority of scholastic volleyball teams are girls' teams, since volleyball was one of the greatest beneficiaries of Title IX expansions over the past forty years. (To learn more about the history, goals, and impact of Title IX, see chapter 34.) Therefore, I will focus primarily on that aspect of the sport, although beach volleyball and boys' teams are certainly an important part of the overall sport as well.

The biggest culprit behind lost playing time in volleyball is ankle injuries. The most serious are subtle fractures and damage to the cartilage, which are often not diagnosed until an X-ray or MRI following several weeks of persistent pain. Because they are generally not catastrophic in nature, many athletes try to play through the pain, believing that the injury will resolve itself. Usually injuries can be treated nonoperatively with bracing and physical therapy. It is important to remember, though, that if the ankle cannot support weight, the player should not return to the game until she is able to balance on the toes of the affected side without pain. Surgery is usually not necessary for ankle injuries in volleyball; however, if an athlete suffers recurrent ankle sprains that have not been resolved by bracing or strength exercises, a physician may consider surgery.

One easy way to keep the ankles flexible and strong is to practice "writing" the alphabet with each foot. Sit in a comfortable position with the legs extended in front. Go through all twenty-six letters with each foot; alternatively, try writing the numbers one through thirty. This helps work the joint in all directions as the toes slowly and deliberately trace the shapes in the air. If desired, attach light ankle weights for more of a workout. Another very simple ankle stretch can be performed by sitting barefooted on the floor with the legs extended straight in front of the body. Slowly point the toes, keeping the heels on the ground, but trying to get the toes as close to touching the ground as possible. Hold for a count of twenty and repeat. The back can either be kept in a straight posture, perpendicular with the floor, or else the stretch can be modified by leaning forward, much as one would when touching the toes, but, instead, use the hands to grasp the ankles or arches of the feet. Either position helps limber up the ankle, and as the joint's flexibility increases, the toes will get closer and closer to touching the ground. Some people with extremely high arches and/or flexible ankles may be able to actually make both the heel and toes touch, but that is not the ultimate goal of the exercise, so long as the tendons and ligaments of the ankle are being stretched gently.

Ankles are certainly not the only joint under stress in volleyball, though. Knees endure a great deal of impact because of spiking and blocking at the net, which subject the joint to repetitive, forceful jumping activities. Patellar tendinitis results when the tendon that connects the kneecap (patella) to the shinbone (tibia) becomes inflamed. Patellar tendon straps are available that can help defer the stress to the joint, but athletes should focus on strength-building and flexibility exercises for long-term knee health. Preseason strength training of the legs will help build up the muscles surrounding the joint, and proper stretching will also keep the knee flexible. Clearly, proper jumping techniques should also be practiced. Whenever possible, avoid locking the knees when coming down from a leap, and land on the balls of your feet and then allow your weight transfer toward your heels, ending in an athletic position.

ACL tears can also plague volleyball players, especially if the athlete lands a jump awkwardly. If the athlete hears or feels a *pop* in her knee, and swelling follows immediately afterward, a physician should be consulted right away, as an MRI will often be required to confirm the injury. Unlike many other sprains and injuries, ACL tears do not heal on their own; reconstructive surgery will be necessary for athletic activity to be resumed. Since recovery and rehabilitation can last anywhere from six to twelve months, athletes should protect their knees through equipment, exercises, and proper technique.

The lower back is another problem area for volleyball players. Muscle or ligament strain can be treated with rest, heat, and gentle stretching, but more serious pain can indicate a herniated spinal disc. If back pain radiates down the leg to cause pain, numbness, tingling, or weakness in the foot or ankle, seek an MRI.

Because volleyball is an overhead hitting sport, the shoulder is also key for volleyball players, especially during serving and spiking. Rotator cuff muscles in the shoulder rarely tear in younger players, but they can become fatigued by overuse. If the pain is persistent, it may be necessary to consult a physician; however, rest and physical therapy are often enough to bring down the irritation. The shoulder may also be injured, or even dislocated, by diving for low balls on a hardwood floor, so athletes should take special care to use proper form.

If bruising appears on the forearms, that may be a sign of incorrect technique. While it is natural that impact with the ball during the game will leave red marks, these should fade quickly and not remain sore to the touch the next day. If a player has visible damage to the skin or blood vessels following a practice or game, she should talk with her coach about ways to adapt her playing style. Bruises (also called contusions) form when capillaries break beneath the skin's surface, causing blood to pool. As you are certainly aware, the body usually does an excellent job of healing the damaged area within a week. However, if a bruise appears exceptionally dark and large, or if the skin underneath feels hard, this may be an indication of deep tissue damage or even injury to the underlying bone and may require medical attention.

Fingers are particularly vulnerable to fractures and dislocations, especially during setting, digging, and blocking, when the ball makes sharp contact with the fingertips. Tendon and ligament tears can also occur if the impact is at an unnatural angle. Because treatment will differ significantly depending on the type of injury, it is important to check with the team's athletic trainer if the finger cannot be bent, straightened, or otherwise moved normally.

The best possible prevention of injuries in volleyball is to focus on proper practice conditions for joint health and to take the necessary steps to help strengthen or reinforce any joint with a history of weakness. For instance, jump training should be conducted on mats or rubberized surfaces rather than on concrete or asphalt. The repeated action of jumping and landing can compound over time. The impact from harder surfaces may wear down the joint in an undetectable way, causing damage or weakness until a more significant injury arises. Similarly, utilizing external support such as ankle braces or taping can significantly strengthen the joint and help prevent it from rolling. Volleyball players should use some sort of padded knee protectors to prevent against contusions or bursitis to the front of their knees from direct contact with the floor. Ideally, athletes should dedicate a portion of practice time to conditioning their lower back, shoulders, and legs under proper supervision. A plan built around a gradual progression will help to ensure that the muscles are gently and progressively strengthened to endure competition.

Chapter 29
Water Polo

It might come as a surprise to see a sport like water polo included alongside such mainstream American sports as football, basketball, and softball. But since the 1990s, water polo has been expanding rapidly in this country as more and more athletes have discovered what an intense workout and fun competition the sport provides. Water polo requires the endurance of swimming, the strength and flexibility of wrestling, the passing strategy of basketball, and the throwing ability of baseball—so it's no wonder that the sport produces some of the most physically fit athletes!

And, just like fielding in baseball or playing defense in basketball, a water polo player is most likely to suffer injury due to repetitive throwing motions that can cause wear and tear on both the elbow and shoulder. This is compounded by the fact that the athlete cannot anchor his body with his legs the way a pitcher might in baseball; the result is an increased risk of fatigue of the shoulder or the upper back, which causes instability when the player cocks back his arm to throw. Studies have shown that an astounding 80 percent of water polo players will face some kind of shoulder pain, which means that the problem is clearly an issue that needs to be addressed. The most effective means of preventing overuse injuries to the shoulder and elbow are to undertake conditioning exercises before the season starts. Workouts that gradually increase in weight and focus primarily on the deltoids, the large, triangular shoulder muscles, will not only strengthen the muscles but will also provide natural stabilization of the ligament, the biceps tendon, and the rotator cuff, which is so crucial to the throwing motion. This can prevent tears in the labrum as well as help guard against more acute injuries such as shoulder dislocation, which may result from player-to-player contact. Also, scapular stabilization exercises should be a mainstay of water polo training. Workouts that also focus on the biceps, triceps, and brachialis will lend extra support to the elbow in addition to arm strength. Both the shoulder and the elbow should be stretched before conditioning, practices, and games, as flexibility is key to avoiding some overuse injuries. For example, the athlete can clasp his hands over his head and, using the shoulder muscles to pull the arms backward slightly, hold that position for a count of ten. Then he can clasp his hands behind his back and gently raise the arms upward for another count of ten. Repeating simple stretches like these three or four times, as well as a full-body warm-up to get the blood flowing, can help prepare the muscles for the rigors they are about to endure.

Core exercises can also help prevent fatigue of the shoulder and upper back and protect against strain to the lumbar discs of the lower back, which can sometimes occur as a result of the twisting and torquing required in evasion and throwing. Water polo requires a lot of trunk rotation and twisting upward from the pelvis, so core-strengthening exercises are essential. A weight machine that is designed to allow "reverse crunches"—that is, using the muscles of the lumbar region to move a weight while leaning backward—can be an excellent way of building up strength in this area and also increasing flexibility.

Treading water for extended periods of time is, of course, a necessary component of water polo, and requires not only a high level of cardiovascular fitness but also strength in the quadriceps muscles and flexibility of the hips and hamstrings. Any athlete complaining of hip pain should rest until the joint has healed, and then focus on developing the hip flexor muscles for a stronger and more efficient kick. The knees may also be a source of pain because of the repetitive motion required to keep the swimmer afloat. Meniscal tears or ligament strain may result from prolonged treading and should be treated with rest and ice until the pain subsides; otherwise the athlete risks irritating the joint further and causing more serious rips or tears to the connective tissue. Any dryland exercises designed to strengthen the muscles surrounding the knee will help to reduce the chance of injury, provided that they are done gradually and with proper caution to not exhaust or overload the joint.

It is also important to note that the pool temperature should be maintained between 77 and 82 degrees Fahrenheit. If the temperature is too low, it can cause the body's temperature to drop and muscles to cramp; too high, and the athlete may become overheated. In either case, the athlete should exit the water until his body temperature regulates. Pools used for competition should have automatic temperature regulation, but if a practice pool skews too far to one temperature extreme or the other, more sensitive athletes may find that their body responds negatively.

Finally, facial injuries can result from the simplest of all causes: unclipped or jagged fingernails and toenails. Make sure that players keep their nails trimmed and neatly filed; it may even be advisable to keep clippers and a waterproof metal emery board in the team's first aid kit. Headgear should always be worn to protect the ears from contact and to help prevent swimmer's ear, a condition resulting from water getting trapped in the ear canal.

If players take care to educate themselves on the rules and are willing to condition properly, water polo can be an excellent way to stay fit, learn teamwork and sportsmanship, and develop a unique and powerful athletic skill set that will serve them well both in and out of the pool.

Chapter 30

Wrestling

It is one of the most ancient sports and one of the most popular sports worldwide. Despite its different varieties, such as Greco-Roman and freestyle (which are both Olympic sports), it is collegiate, or "folkstyle," wrestling that is dominant among high school and college teams.

Collegiate-style wrestling is, without a doubt, the most physical of all youth contact sports. It allows the wrestler to use his legs and his opponent's legs in defense and offense. Athletes remain in extremely close contact with each other throughout the match, with the sole goal of physically forcing one's opponent to the ground. As you might imagine, the potential for certain types of injuries is quite different from other sports.

Perhaps the most fundamental health concern is tied to the athlete's weight management. Because a wrestler has a distinct advantage being at the top of his or her weight class, many athletes hover right at the line. The result is often a last-minute push to drop a few pounds. Every year, it seems, we read another story in the news of a high school wrestler who goes to extreme lengths to "make weight." Several commonly used techniques include intentional starvation, prolonged dehydration, attempting to sweat out the extra water weight through the excessive use of saunas or steam baths, or even more extreme purging methods. These are incredibly dangerous, especially when done repeatedly over the course of a season or if there is some previous unknown health risk, such as a heart condition. A properly controlled diet, preferably overseen by the coach in conjunction with a dietician, is far more effective, sustainable, and healthy in the long term for a wrestler. Nutritional advice should emphasize daily caloric requirements and a balanced diet based on age, body size, growth, and physical activity level.

In an effort to combat weight fluctuations, minimum-weight certification programs have been adopted by most wrestling associations. In these programs, each wrestler must weigh in during the first two weeks of the season so that his or her weight is registered as a kind of marker. Subsequent weigh-ins must not fluctuate more than 7 percent from the initial number.

Parents of wrestlers should be aware of their child's eating and exercise habits. While it may be normal to cut back on food a few days before a weigh-in, eliminating food and water altogether should be strongly discouraged. Parents should also learn to recognize the warning signs of hypoglycemia (low blood sugar), including shakiness, sweating or shivering, dilated pupils, confusion, and heart palpitations. If a wrestler exhibits any of these symptoms, he should be given immediately a glass of fruit juice and a complex carbohydrate such as bread or crackers. As some parents of hypoglycemic children have found, it can even help to squirt a small amount of cake decorating gel between the lips and gums so that the liquefied sugar can be absorbed into the circulation more rapidly.

The risk of injury during practice and competition is also something to be aware of. For example, cauliflower ear isn't just something that boxers talked about in old black-and-white movies. It is caused by severe bruising of the outer ear structure and can occur easily during a struggle on the mat. If the ear cartilage is traumatized, fluid can build up. This may need to be drained and the ear wrapped in a casting material to help it retain a normal shape once the swelling has subsided, although it does not always return to its preinjury appearance. Headgear can help prevent this injury, though it is admittedly difficult to eliminate the risk altogether.

Headgear is also important in avoiding concussions—especially headgear with a frontal pad. The warning signs and latent symptoms of concussions are discussed in greater length in chapter 31, but parents should be aware that a concussion may have occurred even if the athlete retains consciousness after impact to the head. Any wrestler who displays signs of dizziness, confusion, or disorientation after striking his head on the mat should be removed from competition and not allowed to return until he has been evaluated and cleared to do so by a physician.

Mouth guards also help prevent concussions by absorbing some of the impact to the front and sides of the head, and they obviously help protect against tooth and tongue injuries as well. For this reason, it is essential that equipment fit properly and be replaced when it begins to show signs of wear or damage. Wrestlers should never engage in any grappling without their headgear and mouth guards in place.

Even more than the head, however, knees take a lot of impact in wrestling, as this is the body part that hits the mat most often. Prepatellar bursitis is the inflammation of the sac (bursa) located in front of the kneecap (patella), which can cause sharp pain and sometimes swelling. Knee pads designed specifically to prevent or control this condition are strongly recommended. If prepatellar bursitis does develop, it can be treated by an over-the-counter anti-inflammatory medication such as ibuprofen or aspirin, plus ice and rest. Wrestlers should pay special attention to any persistent pain behind the kneecap and alert their coach if it does not diminish, in order to avoid long-term damage to the joint. Rehabilitation after an injury is an important part of preventing further injury, since many injuries result from aggravation of an old injury.

Shoulder injuries are certainly not uncommon in wrestling. A number of wrestling holds can cause shoulder subluxations or even full dislocations. Recurrent neglected shoulder dislocations are far too common in wrestling. Young wrestlers have a tendency to pop their own shoulders back in place (self-reduction) and continue the match. Obviously, those shoulders need surgical attention, and because of the injury's tendency to recur, affected shoulders are very hard to repair or reconstruct surgically. They are often not fixable by arthroscopic techniques and frequently require a more invasive, open operation.

Knee ligament injuries due to twisting the joint from the midline of the body can also occur during wrestling, most commonly to the inside (medial collateral ligament, or MCL) or outside (lateral collateral ligament, or LCL) of the knee. Minor sprains can be treated with RICE therapy (rest, ice, compression, and elevation) and the athlete can return to wrestling once the pain subsides. However, more serious sprains should be examined by a physician to ensure that there is no more serious damage. The best means of preventing ligament injuries in wrestling is to perform leg flexibility exercises diligently, focusing especially on the calf and hamstring muscles. Simple stretches such as toe touches can help to keep the hamstrings limber. Athletes should be careful not to "bounce" when stretching—that is, pushing the body in short bursts to reach farther than the body can hold—as this can cause small tears in the muscles. Instead, athletes should try flexibility stretches both before and after workouts to help gently warm up and cool down the muscles. Strength building in the quadriceps and hamstrings will also help to protect the knee from injury, as will careful supervision and coaching in proper technique.

Perhaps the most serious health risk in high school wrestling has nothing to do with an injury but is instead the risk of infection. Skin infections—most notably MRSA (methicillin-resistant *Staphylococcus aureus*)—have been on the rise in schools over the past decade. As the name implies, MRSA is resistant to most antibiotics, as are many of these so-called superbugs, which can, and have, turned deadly. Even more minor infections, such as ringworm, impetigo, conjunctivitis, and herpes simplex, can spread rapidly through teams due to the skin-to-skin contact that wrestling involves, as well as skin-to-mat contact. A small cut or scrape may not be of much consequence to athletes in other sports, but it can lead to an infection in a wrestler. Any wound should be reported to the coach, trainer, or personal physician as soon as possible so that proper care can be started.

If an athlete shows signs of an infection, a physician should be consulted right away to prescribe the appropriate oral or topical antibiotic to treat the condition. It is important that the wrestler avoid any skin-to-skin contact until the infection is gone. It is fine for the athlete to continue to practice with the team provided that he avoid physical contact with teammates.

To help prevent an infection epidemic on a team, insist upon basic hygiene for all the members, including showers before and after practice, and clean workout clothes each day. The mat must also be cleaned with an antiseptic solution immediately after every practice to keep germs from multiplying.

With a few simple steps to protect themselves, wrestlers can enjoy their sport in safety. Overall health and fitness should be the goal of every youth sports program. The best way to maintain a competitive edge and nurture one's talent is by making responsible and smart choices on a daily basis.

Part 3

A Prescription for Change

Introduction

Once we are aware of the risks, benefits, treatments, and prevention techniques, what is our next move? All the knowledge in the world can't help us if we don't actually take the necessary steps to implement real and lasting change.

The following chapters are my closing thoughts, of sorts, to help readers see the broader picture of youth sports, the changing field of youth sports medicine, and why it is ultimately about more than just producing varsity soccer players or future Olympic gymnasts. It's about what is really going on in the minds of some of the most promising young talent. It's about the current climate and future trajectory of youth sports in America. It's about preparing our kids for life both in sports and in the world.

Chapter 31

Concussions and Emergency Action Plans (EAP)

There are two essential elements to youth sports injury prevention that need to be highlighted: concussions and the need for an emergency action plan.

Turning first to concussions, parents must understand not only what the injury is and its causes but also familiarize themselves with the less commonly recognized warning signs that may result in a missed diagnosis.

Concussion sometimes goes by the more descriptive name of mild traumatic brain injury (MTBI), but it is hard to describe exactly how the injury occurs. Unlike a damaged joint or torn ligament, there is not one clear point of injury; instead, the best way to imagine a concussion is to picture the soft matter of the brain being slammed against the hard bones of the skull—almost like shaking Jell-O in a Tupperware container. When an individual suffers any kind of trauma to the head, such as hard contact with the ground after a fall or a tackle, or being hit in the head with a ball or other piece of equipment, there is a risk that the brain may have suffered trauma that could disrupt normal function.

Warning signs of a concussion are sometimes very easy to spot, such as a loss of consciousness or uneven pupil size. However, these telltale markers need not be present for a concussion to have occurred. In fact, some of the other symptoms are far more common. Following any kind of blow or fall involving the head, the affected athlete should be evaluated for these signs of concussion:

- nausea
- headache
- dizziness
- blurred vision
- double vision
- confusion or disorientation
- slowed reaction time
- problems with balance
- sleepiness or feeling in a fog
- difficulty concentrating
- memory problems
- sensitivity to light or noise

No athlete should be allowed to reenter the game or practice until he or she has been evaluated and cleared to do so by a qualified health professional.

During the first twenty-four to forty-eight hours following a concussion, it is important that the athlete be put under minimal physical and mental stress. This obviously means that he or she should not return to the game or practice, but there are other prohibitions as well. For example, the athlete should not attempt to read or study, nor should he or she type or work on a computer. Movies, video games, and even text messaging should all be avoided until the brain has had a chance to recover. Additionally, heavy or spicy foods, alcohol consumption, and the use of nonsteroidal anti-inflammatory drugs such as aspirin, ibuprofen, and naproxen should all be avoided for fear of worsening bleeding. Injured athletes should avoid driving or operating any other type of machinery. It is safe for the affected person to be given acetaminophen for the pain, to have ice packs applied to the head and neck, to sleep, and to eat light meals. Also, some emerging science shows that 1 gram daily for thirty days of docosahexaenoic acid (DHA) omega-3 may assist the brain in righting itself. The student's teachers should be made aware of what has occurred so that alternative arrangements for tests and assignments may be made if necessary.

Parents should be aware that the effects of a concussion can last up to three weeks. If a concussion is suspected, be on the lookout for any changes in normal behavior such as restlessness, lethargy, disturbed sleep patterns, tearfulness or depression, or other emotional responses that seem inappropriate to the situation. These can all be indicators that the brain has suffered injury and is still trying to repair itself.

All concussions, no matter how mild, are serious and must be treated like the medical emergency that they are. In other words, there is no such thing in concussion lingo as a "ding" anymore. More and more studies are showing the damaging effects of multiple concussions on the long-term mental and physical health of athletes. Recent findings indicate that professional football players with three or more confirmed concussions have a higher risk of neurophysiologic changes in the future. Since a player who is suspected of having suffered a concussion faces a higher risk for a repeat injury if he returns to the game without being examined, an immediate response to a suspected concussion is essential. The team's medical professional may choose to evaluate a player pulled from the game with a suspected concussion, but a CT scan may be recommended for an athlete whose symptoms are especially troubling or severe.

Many states have what are called return-to-play laws designed to protect young athletes who have been diagnosed with concussion or are suspected of having a concussion. These policies restrict when players can return to play following their injury for the sake of protecting the player. I am very proud that the Andrews Institute was instrumental in recently getting such a law passed in the state of Florida. Protecting the long-term health of our children is far more important than the score of a sporting event.

One of the major factors in proper concussion care is simply education. Parents, grandparents, coaches, and athletes alike need to be aware of all of the warning signs of concussion and how to react when such an injury is suspected. I recommend that an emergency action plan (EAP) be put into place for every youth sports team, and that it be laminated and posted in clearly visible locations around the training, practice, and competition facilities so that all parties may be aware of it. Parents and grandparents should make it their responsibility to serve as watchdogs to ensure that an EAP is in place where their young athlete plays or practices.

Emergencies are, unfortunately, an unavoidable part of athletics. Concussions, spinal injuries, cardiac arrest, heat illness, severe asthma attacks, sudden complications from sickle-cell anemia, and other potentially life-threatening situations need to be anticipated in order to maximize the expediency of care in situations where seconds count.

The first step is to ensure that every athlete has undergone a basic physical examination by a qualified physician or nurse-practitioner. Many schools and communities offer free or low-cost clinics and preparticipation programs for students. A program's certified athletic trainers and coaches may also wish to conduct baseline assessments of athletes as well, observing physical symptoms following activities such as a ten-minute run, a ten-minute bike ride, a few sprints, and agility drills or weight training. Such observations can help to identify potential problematic conditions before the child or teen begins training in a more strenuous setting where health concerns could manifest in more serious ways. If a school does not have a certified athletic trainer on staff to help facilitate such efforts, parents and grandparents should get involved. In fact, one of the most important things that parents and grandparents can do for the ultimate health care of their young athletes is to help push for state mandates and funding that all public schools should have a full-time, certified athletic trainer. The athletic trainer is vital for early detection and prevention of athletic injuries and will ensure compliance with EAP guidelines.

For athletes who sustain serious injuries, an EAP should lay out clear guidelines for the identification of symptoms and contain a treatment plan for each situation. It should also clearly indicate where emergency equipment—such as first aid kits, backboards, spinal immobilization units, and automated external defibrillators (AED)—is located. It is extremely important that the AED device receive regular maintenance to ensure that it is in working order and holding a charge. In some places, the local rescue squad checks the AEDs at sporting venues and schools on a monthly basis. Parents and coaches should educate themselves on the proper maintenance procedures and location of the AED at their child's event. It is not enough to simply have the device—if it is not properly charged, it can't save a life. Additionally, it is essential that there are medical personnel on hand who know how to use the device properly.

I would encourage all coaches and parents to get certified in CPR from the American Red Cross. Classes in first aid and AED use are also offered and may spell the difference between life and death. Of course, in an ideal situation, qualified health care professionals will be present to step in should the unthinkable happen; however, a knowledgeable parent or coach may be needed in a pinch.

A copy of the emergency action plan should be sent home with every student-athlete so that parents may review it and be aware of what steps are in place to protect their child in the event of an accident. And, as I stated above, copies of it should be posted permanently in several strategic locations around the practice or competition facility so that everyone is aware of the proper measures. It is normal for people to panic when an emergency arises and react in ways that may not be helpful and could even be dangerous; by planning for each eventuality ahead of time, the incident can come as less of a surprise, and cooler heads may prevail.

Should an injury occur when a parent or guardian is not present and no hospitalization is required, the EAP should stipulate that the affected athlete be sent home with a letter informing his or her parents about what happened. This can be a simple form letter that alerts the parent, for example, that the child may have suffered a concussion that day, and includes a list of signs to watch out for, simple instructions for care, and a note outlining when to contact a health care professional should the athlete's condition change. By keeping parents informed, we can all help to protect young athletes from harm.

Chapter 32
Dynamic Warm-Up Exercises

It is widely accepted that both warming up and cooling down are beneficial for athletes. Raising the body's core temperature, activating muscles, and getting the blood flowing are essential before any physical activity. Slowing down the heart rate, reducing the incidence of muscle soreness, and reducing the effects of lactic acid are all good reasons to cool down. The methods used to prepare the body for aggressive physical activity, however, have evolved over recent years.

Until recently, the accepted method of warming up consisted of light aerobic activity followed by a series of static, or "hold," stretches. The thought was that this helped reduce injuries and improve performance. However, numerous research studies have shown very little to support these concepts. Many studies actually demonstrate a decrease in speed, strength, and power after static stretching. I do support static stretching as a part of rehabilitation protocols, as a postexercise cooldown, and when specifically prescribed by a knowledgeable sports medicine professional. However, static stretching may not be the most beneficial way of preparing an athlete's body before play.

Sports are dynamic in nature, which is why active and dynamic warm-ups are appropriate before playing. I propose taking the athlete through exercises with full pain-free range of motion in a controlled manner. This is especially important because the typical day for young people now tends to be quite sedentary. Even if a child is very active in sports, this does not ensure that he or she has good dynamic body control. Training for fitness, athleticism, and dynamic body control will improve performance and reduce the chance of injury.

Here are some different types of stretching and their definitions:

- **Static stretching:** holding a stretch for longer than a few seconds and up to one minute or more. It can be *active*, where the athlete stretches himself, or *passive*, where a partner stretches the body part for him or her.
- **Dynamic stretching:** functional and/or sports-specific movements that cause an eccentric muscle contraction as to replicate the stress experienced during sports activities. Eccentric contractions occur when the muscle elongates under tension due to a force being greater than the force generated by the muscle.
- **Ballistic stretching:** using momentum to stretch a muscle. When done too aggressively, this may lead to injury. The term is often used synonymously with *dynamic stretching*, but for this purpose is defined above.
- **Proprioceptive neuromuscular facilitation (PNF) stretching:** using a combination of passive or dynamic stretching with isometric contraction.

Dynamic warm-up and dynamic flexibility programs should consist of ten to twenty minutes of movements that get the body ready for the activity that day. A dynamic warm-up should incorporate light "form running," skipping, shuffling, crossover stepping or carioca, and backward running. Dynamic flexibility exercises often consist of a series of stretching activities that are held for a few seconds or less. They can incorporate knee hugs, quad pulls, hamstring soldier kicks, glute stretching, fire hydrant groin stretching, lunge walking, sidelunge walking, "Spiderman," and inchworms. Some examples are shown below. For an example of a full preplay dynamic warm-up and dynamic flexibility program, see illustrations below.

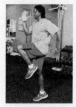 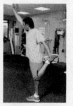 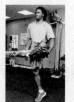

Skipping   Carioca   Quad Pull   Hamstring   Walking Lunge
                                                  Soldier Kick

It is important to start a dynamic or active warm-up with slow and controlled movements. Progress to moderate speed and ultimately into full speed near the end of the warm-up. Overextending a body part is not recommended and can lead to injury, especially in untrained individuals.

Each sport may have specific flexibility needs. Some examples are the sleeper stretch for baseball pitchers; an emphasis on static stretching for dancers and gymnasts, who need to hold poses; latissimus and pectoralis static stretching; gastrocnemius/soleus (calf) static stretching; and active ankle mobility for basketball and volleyball players. Athletes should discuss their specific warm-up needs and goals with their coaches to incorporate the ballistic warm-up techniques that are best for the individual sport.

Chapter 33
Debunking a Few Myths

As I've watched the field of sports medicine grow over the past forty years, I have seen a lot of attitudes toward it change. When I first started practicing, many people were skeptical about an entire branch of medicine dedicated solely to the health of athletes; they tended to trust their general practitioner for everything from a runny nose to tennis elbow. Now, however, people have really opened up to the idea of a physician trained specifically in activity-related injuries, both for diagnosis and treatment as well as prevention. However, there are several prominent misconceptions about the field that I believe need to be addressed in order for people to have a fuller understanding of what sports medicine is and how it can benefit their lives or the lives of their children.

Myth 1: Tommy John surgery will improve pitching performance.

This is one of the most prominent and troubling myths I have ever encountered in my career, and it is absolutely and unequivocally false.

Time after time, I see adolescent pitchers—fourteen to eighteen years old—come to my office complaining of pain and requesting to have this surgery. When we do the diagnostic examinations, however, the scar tissue and tendon damage one would expect to see are simply not there. Pitchers (and their families) often believe that, rather than rehabilitating a sore arm, they should undergo surgery because so many other pitchers have improved their game drastically after the procedure.

I cannot be clearer about this: There is nothing that sports medicine can do for a throwing arm that is better than how the good Lord created it. There is no surgery that enhances performance. It simply does not exist. If the body entered this world whole and healthy, you can never repair something in the body to make it better than its original condition. It's just not possible. Cutting something always makes it weaker. I cannot stress this enough: A healthy pitching arm will always, *always* be more stable and more capable than one that has been operated on.

Yes, it is true that many pitchers do see an upswing in their pitching speeds after undergoing the surgery. The reason for that, however, has nothing to do with a tightening of the ligaments to allow for a greater throwing force, despite what many people believe. *Pitching improves because of the type of reconditioning and physical therapy that the athlete undergoes as he heals from the procedure.* Because he is able to work his arm in a controlled, carefully supervised and monitored environment, he avoids the damaging and fatiguing risks of practice. By working out one-on-one with a qualified trainer, he develops habits and techniques that maximize his natural talent and nurture his own hurling style. The other aspect of performance improvements is related to age, maturity, and natural development of an immature body. One must also realize that baseball is a "developmental sport." Parents need to understand that young adolescent throwers develop differently—some at an early age, while others are late bloomers. Ironically, it is these late bloomers who often become the best athletes as they mature. Therefore, parents should be aware of their perspective and be patient with their young, developing athlete. Any young pitcher considering Tommy John surgery in the hopes of improving his performance should take this to heart and look for a pitching coach instead of a scalpel-wielding surgeon.

Myth 2: Certain other orthopedic surgeries will actually increase overall joint capabilities and, ultimately, performance.

No, they won't. See Myth 1. Read it twice.

Myth 3: There is sufficient medical oversight in scholastic athletic leagues.

Unfortunately, this is woefully untrue, and many parents don't realize how underresourced the medical care is for their child's team until they're facing an injured child and a dearth of options.

In fact, the medical resources offered to athletes can be described best as an inverted pyramid. At the top, the professional level, is the widest part. Every possible type of care for treating injuries is available: from world-class doctors, surgeons, therapists, and athletic trainers, to chiropractors and therapeutic masseuses, to state-of-the-art diagnostic and rehabilitation equipment. The upside-down pyramid narrows a bit at the college level, but there are still great doctors, surgeons, and specialized athletic trainers and treatment options such as whirlpools and ice baths. At the high school level, general athletic trainers are usually not available for all of the sports, and there are not always emergency medical teams present at games and competitions. Parents are usually responsible for getting their child to a doctor for any injury not requiring a rescue squad. As the inverted pyramid reaches its peak at the junior high or middle school level, there is almost no care provided whatsoever. Sometimes there is an interested parent with a medical background or just a volunteer on the sidelines with a first aid kit.

The irony, of course, is that if more medical resources were made available to children when they were younger, the need for such extensive treatment options at the professional level would greatly decrease because the athletes would already know how to protect their bodies and recover from injuries, and they would not be working around the ambient pain from older injuries. The upside-down medical care for athletes should be turned around to favor the young who are, unfortunately, more vulnerable to injury due to their developing bodies.

Therefore, parents and coaches alike should work to provide greater medical oversight for youth leagues. Middle school and high school athletic trainers do wonderful work, but they are often stretched thin looking after a half dozen sports teams at once. Any support that they can be offered in terms of funding, facilities and equipment, or team expansion would make a major difference in the level of care they are able to offer each student-athlete. One of the major goals of the American Orthopaedic Society for Sports Medicine's STOP Sports Injuries program is to mandate certified athletic trainers in all public schools. If parents and grandparents are looking for a way to get involved in their community, this is one great place to help by showing their support for such initiatives.

Myth 4: No pain, no gain.

Don't believe the old adage "No pain, no gain." That's simply not true. Pain exists for a reason: to warn our bodies when something is wrong. Too often, coaches and/or parents put it into their young players' heads that they need to "play through the pain," so kids accept that hurting is just part of the game. This idea is also promoted by "motivational" quotations on T-shirts and signs posted around weight rooms that say things such as "Pain is weakness leaving the body."

Utter nonsense.

Of course, there is going to be some discomfort when getting into peak physical shape. This pain is necessary as the muscles break down to rebuild themselves stronger and more resilient than before. But, as I said in chapter 4, the goal is to be *better* each day, not worse. It's one thing to feel some soreness in the muscles a day or two after a workout, but it's something entirely different to be in so much pain that normal movement isn't possible. The problem is realizing the difference between normal soreness and pain.

After a good workout, an athlete should feel exhausted but exhilarated, not fatigued and hurting. Think about how you feel after completing a major project or presentation for work, when you know you did a fantastic job. You sink into a chair, so relieved that it's over and completely wiped out by all you did to prepare—but you're also grinning from ear to ear because you know that you absolutely did your best and really accomplished something great. That's the kind of feeling that should follow a practice or a game. Of course, there will be tough days and even tougher losses, so the grin won't always be there. But the idea is the same: The athlete should always feel as if he or she just accomplished something great that is moving him or her toward a goal. There should never be a feeling of dread for the next day because of the pain it will bring the body, or grimacing because of the unbearable soreness that is plaguing a joint, muscle, or bone. Young athletes should recognize the difference between soreness that gets better with properly executed warm-ups versus pain that gets worse with further participation.

To put it bluntly, no child or teen should ever play with pain. Period. If the body is alerting the brain that something is wrong, the brain should listen. Parents, coaches, and players all need to remember that nothing is more important than the athlete's health.

Myth 5: The earlier a child begins a sport and the more he or she practices, the better the chances are for a scholarship or professional career.

The media loves to highlight the human interest side of sports phenoms. When stories come out about players with unbelievable talent who were showing promise by the age of five, like golfer Tiger Woods, I always cringe a little. There are, of course, some young phenoms who can handle that kind of stress and workload—but their genetic makeup is one in a million! Yes, those stories are interesting, and I am always happy for anyone who is able to make his or her dream of becoming a pro athlete come true. But when I hear about hours spent on the links or in the pool or on the court—when the child is elementary school–aged—I want to pull my hair out. The majority of parents and coaches will hear the same stories and not think twice about it, but, unfortunately, there are others who will view it as a kind of call to action and will begin pushing their child even harder. Some do it because they want the child to earn a scholarship to college, others because they see a big professional contract in the child's future, and others simply because the parents are living vicariously through the child and want him or her to have all the opportunities that they never had. But whatever the motivation is, the end result is almost inevitably the same: The child will get burned out or, worse yet, suffer a traumatic or overuse injury that will haunt him the rest of his life. Statistics show that young athletes who are subjected to extreme specialization and/or professionalism tend to drop out by the age of thirteen.

Some sports and activities are especially prone to this kind of involvement from a young age, such as tennis, figure skating, gymnastics, and dance. Because of the sophisticated techniques required to compete at the highest levels, parents often believe erroneously that their child will be at a disadvantage if he or she is not enrolled in classes by the age of five or six. By the time the child has reached middle school age, he or she is often committed to four or five hours a day of practice. While I am certainly an advocate of organized sports, this level of intensity at such a young age is neither healthy nor beneficial to the child's overall health and long-term career prospects. There is nothing wrong with a once-a-week dance class or a weekend soccer league for an elementary school–aged child, but the vast majority of their activity time should be left unscheduled for free play. Not only does that help to stimulate imagination, as they invent their own games and develop active hobbies and interests, but it also cuts down on the risk of overuse injuries because, unlike in a developmental sports program, a young child will not repeat a movement over and over again if it hurts. Variance in motion is far more beneficial to a child than concentrated and repetitive instruction at a young age.

There is nothing wrong with wanting to give your child an advantage. But please, be smart about how you pursue it. I would recommend that parents allow kids to just be kids at least part of the time. When they are healthy teenagers and young adults with an active future ahead of them, you'll be very glad that you did.

Myth 6: Fast-pitch softball, with its windmill delivery, can't produce injuries to the thrower's shoulder or elbow.

There is a common belief that throwing underhand is a natural way to keep the player safe from injury, but this definitely is not true. I have even heard TV commentators make this erroneous statement recently. Unfortunately, my fellow sports medicine physicians and I are seeing more and more young softball pitchers coming into our offices with throwing-arm injuries to both the shoulder and the elbow. The repeated movement and velocity of pitches thrown, even in the windmill style, are now even tearing the "Tommy John ligament," resulting in a UCL injury. Pitching limits matter in softball as much as they do in baseball.

Myth 7: The sooner the problem can be diagnosed, the sooner the athlete can return to the game.

Sometimes the problem faced by young athletes is not an injury at all—it's burnout. And when that is the diagnosis, there isn't much that a doctor can do to make the child want to return to the field or the court.

I see it all the time: A young person comes in with his or her family, complaining of a certain type of pain, and the symptoms are usually a textbook description of the suspected diagnosis. And yet, when I conduct the exam, I find little evidence of an injury. Still, the parents insist that something is wrong; in fact, it is the parents who are doing most of the talking. The child often sits on the examination table, head hanging down, while the parents go on and on about their concern for how this pain might negatively impact their child's incredible talent and career potential.

In cases like that, I will often ask the parents to step out of the room, and then I will talk with the young man or young woman one-on-one about what is really going on and what he or she is really feeling. It's amazing how many times I hear, "To be honest, Doctor, I'm just tired of practicing my sport, but I don't know how to tell my parents I want to quit." Kids are smart. Despite how much they may kick and scream while doing a research paper for history class, they really do know how to research a topic, and most kids who are suffering have done their homework. They recognize that their parents or coaches or even siblings might not react well to the news that they don't want a future in the sport, so they read up on injuries that would force them to take some time off. They know the causes, they know the symptoms, they know the right complaint to get them out of the starting lineup and into the doctor's office—anything for a break. *And I don't blame them.* After all, who wants to live someone else's dream? Especially when that dream occupies several hours each day or dominates every weekend?

Surveys taken of young athletes indicate that more than 40 percent said they felt pressure from their parents to play. Other studies have shown that 70 to 80 percent of children involved in organized sports will drop out by the age of thirteen, and the most commonly reported reasons were overuse injuries and too much pressure from parents, peers, and/or coaches. The problem is that the majority of the kids who do quit a sport will not take up another organized activity in its place. Not only does this pose a risk for their physical fitness, but it also puts them at much higher risk for getting into trouble in and out of school. Organized sports help to keep kids occupied in positive, healthy ways. That is why playing multiple sports with appropriate time off is so important.

It is also tremendously important for parents to recognize the signs of burnout in their child. If an athlete who was once enthusiastic about going to practice suddenly begins making excuses or acting reluctant, it might be time to sit down and have a heart-to-heart. Maybe the lack of excitement is stemming from something else entirely, but just letting your child know that your love for him or her is not tied to his or her participation or success in a sport (or anything else) is essential to building a strong relationship.

Chapter 34
Title IX and Youth Sports

"No person in the United States shall, on the basis of sex, be excluded from participation in, be denied the benefits of, or be subjected to discrimination under any education program or activity receiving federal financial assistance."

Title IX of the Education Amendments of 1972, itself an amendment of the Civil Rights Act of 1964, has done more to change the face of high school and college sports—and by extension, sports medicine—than any other piece of legislation in American history. For this reason alone, I believe it is essential that athletes and parents educate themselves on its requirements and boundaries.

Interestingly, there was no mention whatsoever of athletics in the original act; however, Title IX has since become synonymous with women's athletic opportunities because it mandated gender equality in terms of funding, recruitment, and facilities for women's sports. There is no question that it has been a tremendous boon for young women across the country, but it is not without controversy, either. I think it is important for parents to be aware of the basic tenets of the law and to be willing to fight for their child's rights when participating in an organized sport, whatever their child's gender.

216

It would be nearly impossible to chronicle the entire timeline and amendments to Title IX, and rather confusing to trace every last measure and countermeasure concerning it. It was a groundbreaking piece of legislation that continues to evolve over time. What is important is the history leading up to the legislation, the ways in which it has been implemented, and the impact it has made.

The goal of the Civil Rights Act of 1964 was to end legalized discrimination against any citizen on the basis of race, ethnicity, or national origin. By extension, women's rights were also promoted, with an eye toward workplace equality and educational opportunities, as discrimination based on gender preferences for hiring, promotions, salary, and admissions was still rampant in many industries and institutions.

In 1969, a woman named Bernice Sandler filed a complaint against the University of Maryland claiming that female employees were being replaced by male employees for no demonstrable reason except for the difference in gender—not on the basis of superior qualifications, skills, or job performance. As the legal matter grew, more complaints were filed against universities and colleges nationwide, citing the nondiscrimination goals of the Civil Rights Act as the legal basis for the cases. Protesters argued that these institutions were accepting federal funding through loans, tuition assistance, and several other avenues of support, and this officially sanctioned discrimination was in direct violation of the legislation. As a result, institutions of higher learning were scrutinized not only for their affirmative action policies but also for their practices toward women.

It was not until three years after Title IX was originally passed in 1972, however, that its impact on women's sports became evident. In 1975, the US Department of Health, Education, and Welfare (which no longer exists in that form) issued its official rulings on how colleges and universities would need to take steps to ensure that there was gender equality within their athletic programs as well as in their classrooms and offices. In subsequent years, several attempts were made to block the measures, including the NCAA's push to have Title IX's application to college athletics deemed illegal. Opponents argued that men's sports traditionally produced far more revenue than women's sports, both in ticket sales and merchandising. The fear was that funds diverted away from these high-grossing sports would significantly hurt the schools financially, especially since the profits generated by athletic programs are generally shared university-wide by academic and research departments as well as sports programs.

Clarification and refinement of institutional requirements and responsibilities continued for the next two decades until the Equity in Athletics Disclosure Act of 1994 laid out the current standards for compliance. In an effort to track progress, schools are now required to divulge their budgets for coaching staff salaries, recruiting, scholarships, and other expenditures; additionally, the roster counts for each men's and women's team must be made public as well.

Compliance is generally measured through what is commonly called the "three-part test." The university must demonstrate that it is meeting or exceeding one or more of the following stipulations:

1. Athletic scholarships are offered in proportion to the school's gender composition. For example, if a school is 52 percent female, then 52 percent of its scholarships must be made available to female athletes.

2. The school can demonstrate that it is continuing to expand athletic opportunities for female athletes, and has a history of doing so.

3. Athletic opportunities are offered in proportion to gender interest. In other words, while there need not be a female equivalent for every male sport and vice versa (female football or male synchronized swimming is not required), there must be an equal number of athletic opportunities made available to both genders through a variety of sports.

The Impact

These efforts have made a considerable difference in the athletic landscape at high schools and colleges. Although the compliance tests took a number of years to evolve, there is a clear connection from the start of Title IX's implementation to the rapid growth of women's sports.

In 1971, the year before the Title IX amendment was passed, participation in women's sports at the university level was around 25,000 nationwide. After President Richard Nixon signed Title IX into law in 1972, female participation began to grow exponentially; now more than 110,000 women participate in intercollegiate sports each year, and the number keeps climbing. Today 98.8 percent of colleges and universities have a women's basketball team; almost as many offer volleyball and soccer. Women's cross-country and softball are represented at more than 89 percent of schools as well. Shifting gender mores, coupled with increased athletic opportunities for young women, meant that Title IX was succeeding. For this, I heartily applaud the amendment and the doors it has opened for aspiring female athletes.

However, for all of the positive changes that Title IX has brought, there have also been some unforeseen negative consequences. Along with this rapid growth in women's sports comes a rapid escalation of female injuries. In some of the women's cutting sports, there is a five- to seven-fold ACL injury rate compared to the same sport for men. There have been other unforeseen consequences as well. Many men's sports have been dialed back to create more opportunities for women. In the fifteen years between 1987 and 2002, more than one thousand men's sports teams were eliminated across the country, while the number of women's sports teams continued to rise, and the trend continues. The reason is that there is just not enough funding to support all of the preexisting male teams *and* expand the athletic offerings for women to achieve equality. Instead, many schools are finding it is much easier to cut the number of male sports to make the number of women's programs match. Some of the sports impacted the most are wrestling, swimming, and track; however, baseball programs have become increasingly threatened as well.

This unforeseen side effect is a tragedy for American scholastic sports. While no one can argue against the importance of allowing young women an equal chance to participate and succeed, it should not be done at the expense of existing opportunities for young men. One of the biggest hurdles created by Title IX is that it does not always take into account varying degrees of *interest* in sports; that is, while schools seek to have a percentage of scholarships and other resources available equal to each gender's population within the student body, it does not take into account the fact that male participation and interest in athletics tends to be higher across the board. Of course, it could be argued that this is a chicken-and-egg scenario: that women's interest would be equally high if they had not historically faced discriminatory funding for their sports programs. But the fact remains that boys' sports should not be punished as we seek to grow girls' sports. If the ultimate goal is to increase participation and healthy, active lifestyles across the board, we should not be doing so by eliminating opportunities.

These cuts are not just threats; they are very real, and they are still happening. More than 180 men's collegiate cross country teams and 180 indoor track teams have been dropped. Nearly as many golf teams and tennis teams have both also been eliminated from schools. Rowing, swimming, wrestling, and outdoor track have also been abolished at many schools. I encourage anyone concerned to get involved. Ask questions, make phone calls, learn about the school's Title IX compliance status and what that might mean for existing sports. Get involved with your favorite program however you can, whether through joining the boosters, volunteering with time or resources, or simply by showing up at games and being a vocal supporter. If you know that a school's track or tennis team is on the proverbial chopping block, write letters to the administration expressing your objections.

Just as it is up to parents to protect their children's bodies and safeguard them from overuse injuries, it is also up to parents to fight back against unfair cuts to sports programs—no matter the gender of the child or the team facing elimination. Discrimination has no place in sports, whether against women's programs or men's. By rolling up our sleeves and showing the administrations that there are talented, motivated athletes who want to represent their school in competition—and that there are fans who will support them—hopefully we can keep doors open for *everyone* who wants a chance to compete.

Chapter 35
The Future of Sports Medicine

When the National Athletic Trainers' Association was founded in Kansas City, Missouri, in 1950, it boasted approximately 125 members. The main topics of discussion at the first conference were "Charley Horses" and "Courtesy to Visiting Teams." Oh, how times have changed. Today there are almost thirty-three thousand members, and the conference topics range from advanced surgical techniques to advances in medicine that sound like something straight out of science fiction. But what does this mean for the next generation of athletes?

When I speak about this topic at conferences around the country, it is humbling to consider the broad spectrum of health care professionals in the room. Many are older physicians like me, trained by the men and women who were the original pioneers in the field of modern sports medicine. We benefited from their hard-fought battles to legitimize sports medicine, and we also rode the wave of excitement in the 1970s when the field introduced arthroscopic surgery. We all stand on the shoulder of those early giants. The ability to insert an endoscopic camera into the body to inspect damage to cartilage, tendons, ligaments, and other soft tissues gave us a window to the body that, previously, only exploratory surgery could offer. Thanks to that advancement, it was possible to develop minimally invasive surgical methods that reduced the amount of trauma to the joint, decreased the length and intensity of recovery time, and maintained the integrity of the joint. I see the current crop of physicians who are now rising to the top of the field, having learned current arthroscopic surgery techniques as well as having the imagination to envision what else might be possible in the future as the boundaries of science are pushed to new limits.

Finally, I see the medical students, residents, and newly minted sports physicians who are just now entering our field where revolutionary techniques are standard practice. No longer is it mere speculation that genes might hold the key to faster recovery, or that tissues could be grown in labs to replace damaged tendons, ligaments, or cartilage. These options, while still cutting edge, are a very real part of their experience, knowledge, and medical philosophy. What was once a crazy idea—like the arthroscope—is now a routine treatment option for patients and has become the standard in a number of other surgical disciplines. And it is the youngest athletes today—the Little League players and the pee-wee soccer tykes—who will benefit. Though, of course, our ultimate hope is that they will never face an injury so severe that medical intervention will be required at all. It is an exciting time for sports medicine as the older generation passes the torch to a younger one on the edge of its own revolution.

I'd like to speak briefly about some of the emerging new methods in sports medicine that exist today, explaining briefly what each one involves and what it can (and can't) do to help the human body repair itself. It is important to stipulate that these advancements are all focused on aiding the healing process, *not* on enhancing performance. Orthopedic researchers are not looking for a way to create a superhuman. And, as I mentioned earlier, the body is a pretty amazing feat of engineering; you can't do much to improve this masterfully designed machine. No surgery can enhance performance. At best it can restore it. But some emerging methods in sports medicine today have revolutionized the healing process as we know it. Let's look at a few of the most promising advancements.

Biologics utilize the body's own natural components for healing.

They are now being used to treat a wide variety of medical issues. One of the most promising area of biologics treatment is gene therapy. Gene therapy is the manipulation of the body's DNA to treat, combat, and heal damage caused by illness, injury, or gene mutation. While most clinical trials have focused on gene therapy as a means of helping the body combat single-gene genetic diseases such as sickle-cell anemia and cystic fibrosis, as well as certain forms of cancer, it is now also showing promise as a means of controlling viruses such as the human immunodeficiency virus (HIV). Gene therapy has potential applications in sports medicine as a means of regenerating damaged tissue. By applying genetic codes to specific proteins, it is possible to expand their healing. This will allow damaged tissues to return to a state closer to their preinjury strength.

Tissue engineering, a technique that, theoretically, will work in tandem with gene therapy, bolsters the cells' ability to regenerate and reproduce, allowing for new tissue to grow where it otherwise might be stunted. This is especially exciting when one considers the challenges of repairing ACL tears, which requires a very invasive surgical procedure followed by many months of recovery and rehabilitation. If the body is able to participate more fully in the repair process, this can greatly reduce the amount of time that patients would spend off their feet postsurgery.

Blood platelets, which are integral to allowing our blood to clot, contribute to all aspects of healing. Their growth factors are necessary to signal other cells, such as stem cells, how to differentiate along a cell line in order to replace or repair damaged cartilage, bone, muscle, or tendon cells. We are now able to concentrate the amount of platelets from a blood sample and then inject or implant those platelets into whatever type of tissue we are trying to heal. This process has been shown to repair and rehabilitate many common injuries that we treat in sports medicine. PRP (platelet-rich plasma) has a successful history in oral surgery and veterinary medicine. The composition of the PRP—higher platelet concentrations versus lower concentrations, the presence or absence of white cells—and the use of platelet activators are all questions that need to be answered with further research in order to validate PRP's use in sports medicine. PRP has justifiably received a great deal of attention in sports medicine, as many athletes have sought it for injured joints, muscles, and bones, and arthritic pain or swelling from older injuries.

Although stem cell research is a highly controversial subject, it has great potential for the healing process. Stem cells are cells that can turn into, or differentiate into, a particular cell such as bone, cartilage, nerve, or muscle, depending on what growth factors are present and the environment the stem cell is in. Stem cells are obtained from various means, such as from a patient's bone marrow, fat cells, blood, and, the most controversial source, embryos. Stem cells can also be obtained from a donor mother's placenta after birth. It is possible to collect stem cells and then cryopreserve (freeze) them through biobanking, to be used at a later date. These stem cells can then be thawed and used to grow in specific ways. We can also culture these cells in the lab to treat an injury. However, the US Food and Drug Administration (FDA) does not allow the culturing of stem cells in the United States to be used for treatment of any kind. For athletes, these cells can mean a potential source for regrowing ligaments, tendons, cartilage, and even muscle tissue that may be damaged beyond the point of surgical repair. They may one day render surgery unnecessary. What were once career-ending injuries may now be fixed and, with physical therapy and careful rehabilitation, the player may once again have a full range of motion in an injured joint. This field is in its infancy, though, and will require more research to figure out how stem cells are used most effectively to treat musculoskeletal injuries.

Outside of the field of biologics, there are advancements that have major implications for orthopedics as well. Robotic surgery, for example, can potentially change the way that doctors can treat patients by enabling them to carry out minimally invasive procedures with even less trauma to the body and—even more exciting—perform surgery without needing to be physically present. By controlling the surgical implements via computer, a surgeon who has a connected clinic could complete an operation on a patient anywhere in the world. For patients in developing countries who need specialized care, this news is tremendous; instead of paying exorbitant fees to travel thousands of miles, one day people may be able to access the treatment they need at their own local clinic.

These changes, as well as new improvements and developments on existing instruments, are opening up a whole new world of possibilities for orthopedists and athletes alike. As the means of treating injuries become more and more refined, and the healing process accelerated and enhanced, athletes will have greater opportunities than ever to continue working toward their goals. Though our primary goal, first and foremost, is to *prevent* injuries, we have never before been better equipped to treat them, thanks to today's cutting-edge medical advancements.

Part 4

Concluding Remarks

Chapter 36
Adventures in Medicine

Although it may seem totally unrelated to youth sports injury prevention, I thought I'd share a little bit about some of the wild, unbelievable experiences I've had over the course of my career, so that people don't get the wrong idea about me—that I'm some overly cautious, kids-should-wear-helmets-at-all-times-and-live-in-a-bubble kind of guy. I'm not. I love to pursue adventure and enjoy an adrenaline rush just as much as anyone. I just want kids' bodies to be protected so that they have the ability to seek adventure in their own lives when it comes knocking, too. I've been fortunate enough that my work in sports medicine has opened doors for my family and me to enjoy some very rewarding and unusual experiences. By keeping their own bodies healthy, today's generation of young people will be ready for whatever doors open for them.

Doctor to a Prince

It was the early 1980s, and I was at the International Arthroscopy Association conference at the Southampton Princess hotel in Bermuda. I had been invited as a guest speaker on arthroscopic surgery in sports medicine, and after my talk, a group of us went over to the hotel bar to chat a while longer. I happened to notice a Middle Eastern man sitting by himself, and I felt bad for his loneliness, as everyone else was attending the conference with their family and friends. This poor guy was all alone, and it showed. I struck up a conversation with him, and it turned out that he was Dr. Mazen Mrad, the head orthopedic surgeon at the military hospital in Riyadh, Saudi Arabia.

His English was impeccable, which made sense because he had studied in London after moving from his native Lebanon, and then practiced medicine in Saudi Arabia. I really enjoyed talking with him, and we traded contact information. Not long afterward, I heard from him again, this time asking if he could bring a patient to the clinic where Dr. Hughston and I worked in Columbus, Georgia. But it wasn't just any patient; it was a member of the Saudi royal family who wanted to have his knee operated on. He was a middle-aged man who had torn his ACL, and the pain was preventing him from pursuing his favorite pastimes of mountain climbing and big game hunting.

I agreed to perform the surgery, and thus began a relationship with the royal family that extended to many years of orthopedic care for many of its members as well as for a number of Saudi athletes. That first royal patient I treated did not want to be seen back home walking with a limp, so he and his entire entourage needed a place to stay. I happened to have a second home that I was trying to sell at the time, so I made that available to him. But it simply wasn't large enough to house him and all of his people. So they made an enormous offer to rent the house next door as well. The owners were friends of mine and decided it would be worth the inconvenience, so they lived in an apartment for six months while the Saudi family used their home as a kind of auxiliary place. My wife, Jenelle, and I would be invited over for dinner several times a week, and we learned that they always used the neighbors' house for cooking and our house for serving. The problem was that at one point, the cooks accidentally set fire to the kitchen of the rented house; the blaze spread to the rest of the structure and almost gutted the home.

In all, between the family, servants, and cooks, there were nearly two hundred people. Obviously, they couldn't all fit in even the two houses, so the rest of the party lived in various places all over Columbus and would trek over to the two main houses each day.

The town was reeling from such a huge influx of exotic faces. No one could get lamb at any grocery store or restaurant because the Saudi cooks bought it all up. In fact, there were so many members of the entourage that the lamb supply was affected all the way to Atlanta. Also, every week the family would rent a Greyhound bus, and all of the women and children would make the hundred-mile trip to Atlanta and back, with the storage holds of the bus absolutely crammed full of everything you could imagine: clothes, shoes, purses, furniture, home décor items, and countless other packages. When it came time for everything to be shipped back to Saudi Arabia, it cost a small fortune to air freight it all home. In the meantime, some of the men were traveling around the country taking advantage of the hunting opportunities. It was just such a completely different cultural experience for both us and them.

Meanwhile, Dr. Mrad, the doctor I had met in Bermuda, was able to obtain a fellowship with me at the Hughston Clinic. He eventually became the orthopedic surgeon to the Saudi royal family and the personal surgeon of Prince Sultan bin Abdel Aziz Al Saud, who was then the minister of defense and later became crown prince before he passed away in 2011. We also had a few other extremely high-ranking royals travel to Columbus for surgery, and later to Birmingham. In fact, when Prince Sultan came to Birmingham, he brought an entourage of nearly eight hundred people; but none of them had nearly as long or as memorable a stay as the very first prince we treated.

But that began an interesting chapter in my life, during the late 1980s and 1990s, when we expanded to have a clinic in Birmingham, Alabama, as well as in Columbus. I was working both clinics Monday through Thursday; then on some weekends, I would fly to Saudi Arabia on Fridays to help with exams and surgeries over there. I'd fly back Sunday night to Monday morning and be available for appointments and house calls in the States by Monday afternoon. I must have made close to twenty-five of those trips, doing my best to sleep as much as I could on the plane rides. The demand for ACL surgeries was unbelievable. There was a waiting list of nearly two thousand athletes for the procedure, most of whom were soccer players. Eventually, the Saudi government agreed to pay for the athletes' transportation and visa fees to come over to our clinic—three or four of them at a time, with their families—and I'd do the surgery and get them started on rehabilitation. It was easier than for me to fly over there so much; plus, they all seemed to love visiting the United States and taking advantage of our shopping. Sometimes they would book an entire hotel and make it a huge event.

Another time, after I was flown into the country to perform surgery and my plane was sitting on the tarmac waiting to take off for home, a fleet of cars pulled up and ordered us off the aircraft. It was the middle of the night, and I had no idea how I was going to make it back to Birmingham in time for my Monday appointments, but I was told that I needed to examine the knee of one of the princesses—and it was clear that saying no was not really an option. I met with the young woman and checked out the joint; then my assistant and I were put on one of the royal family's private jets and flown directly back to London, where we were able to catch a flight to New York and then back to Birmingham in time to meet with my patients there. It was a surreal experience, seeing the almost limitless power and resources of the ruling family.

We had a great relationship with those folks, though. Jenelle would make the trip with me as often as she could, and she really got to be good friends with some of the families. They lavished her with expensive gifts that were not expected but greatly appreciated. I experienced some things a boy from Louisiana never would have dreamed of, such as milking a camel in the middle of the desert! Another prince had a four-hundred-foot ship that he sailed to the Bahamas while he recuperated after I'd operated on his shoulder in Birmingham. I would fly back and forth to check on his progress using a seaplane. It was pretty incredible.

Of course, 9/11 put a stop to all of that because the visas were not as readily available, and travel became much more difficult. But it sure was fascinating and exciting while it lasted, and I hope I was able to help a lot of people in Saudi Arabia, both through the surgeries and treatments I was able to offer and in helping Dr. Mrad get orthopedic surgery more firmly established in the country.

Learning to Sail

I got hooked on sailing while I was in medical school, thanks to a buddy of mine named Chip. He'd been an ensign at the US Naval Academy but got kicked out for sneaking out of the barracks and pulling a big prank on the Army team the night before their football matchup: He wrote "Beat Army" across the bow of the visiting Army ship. He was from Louisiana originally, so he went back to pursue a degree in medicine, and the two of us became fast friends while we were both working through our program at LSU. We would go hunting sometimes, talk about sailing on Lake Ponchartrain, or just look for ways to blow off some steam on the days we were cooped up in the cadaver labs.

One of those ways was to rush out to the racetrack at the fairgrounds during lunch. We had just enough time to bet the first race and the daily double before dashing back to make it to the cadaver lab on time. The head of housekeeping for the medical school at the time also worked as a bookie, so we'd place bets with him if we couldn't make the event in person; some days we'd finish a dissection early so we could head out to the racetrack for the last race of the day. The races were such a contrast to the serious, methodical work in school that it was just a great way for us to separate ourselves from the hours and hours of sensitive and meticulous work that lay on either side of our breaks.

One day, we were both pretty broke—just a dollar and a handful of change between the two of us. We scraped it together to lay down a $2 bet on a horse named Tom's Gamble. He had the longest odds of any horse in the last race on a muddy track, and the name just seemed too perfect for us not to put our last couple of bucks on him. It was a stormy, rainy, awful day. Everyone was miserable, including most of the horses. When the gates opened, all the other horses looked old, tired, and cranky to be outside in such weather, but Tom's Gamble took off like an absolute bullet and never slowed. He won by a dozen lengths, and Chip and I were screaming our heads off. It was absolutely incredible; we won something like $250 on our $2 bet.

Not long before, a huge hurricane had blown through New Orleans and sunk a number of boats moored at the lakefront marina. We took our $250 winnings and headed down to the Southern Yacht Club, where we saw an ad posted on the bulletin board. For $200, you could buy the sails to a Snipe, the same kind of racing dinghy used by the US Olympic sailing team. The deal was, if you bought the sails, the owner would tell you where the boat had gone down so you could salvage it, since he wasn't interested in raising and repairing it himself. The seller's house was right down the street, so we marched there, handed over our money, got the boat's location, and went to work. We strapped on aqua tanks and dove down to pull that darn thing up—which is a whole other adventure in itself—and then spent the entirety of the next vacation from medical school at Chip's home in Morgan City, Louisiana, repairing and fiberglassing that wooden boat with an eye toward racing it.

Now, I had been brought up on small lakes, but Chip had been in the Navy, so I could only assume that he had at least a rudimentary nautical knowledge. I was wrong. He was every bit as clueless as I was, so we ended up buying some really basic Dell paperback called *Learning to Sail,* or something like that, and learned everything we could. Then we drove the boat down to the lake, put it in the water, and learned the rest by trial and error. We eventually sold that first boat, salvaged another, and kept it up until, when we were seniors in medical school, we had a forty-foot wooden racing sailboat.

At that time, there was what was called the Sugar Bowl Regatta, which hosted a sailing expo each year around Christmastime. Ted Turner, the future media mogul, was just getting to be a big-shot name and was very into sailing. He had already won an America's Cup and now entered the race with a Cal forty-footer—just about the most top-of-the-line, unbelievably expensive boat available at the time. Chip and I joined in, too. I mean, we weren't officially registered, but we raced alongside everyone else, and, wouldn't you know it, we beat Turner and his bottomless wallet in a boat that we'd refurbished ourselves. It was one of the best feelings in the world!

I spent a little time studying in San Francisco after medical school and bought a boat so I could live on the water in San Francisco Bay and race while I was out there. I just loved the combination of skill, athleticism, and luck that sailing provided, plus the challenge of racing was great for my competitive side. I would eventually race all over the world, including representing the United States in the Sardinia Cup and a number of fifty-foot association championship races.

America's Cup

My journey to the America's Cup was kind of born out of that Sugar Bowl Regatta race. Ted Turner won the Southern Ocean Racing Conference, a six-week sailing race around Florida and down to the Bahamas, and I decided that if I'd beaten him once, I could do it again. So I worked on a forty-three-footer up in Connecticut, and even though my team was made up mostly of self-taught sailors like me, we somehow managed to hit it just perfectly and ended up winning the race—three times. In fact, we still hold the records for the Miami-to-Nassau race, breaking a fifty-five-year-old record in the process. One of my sailboats, which I had made in Sydney, Australia, won the fifty-foot World Cup Championship and was rated by *Sail* magazine as the top offshore racer in the last one hundred years.

Beyond this, I had always dreamed of being involved in the America's Cup but never really thought it would be possible. In 1992, I got to be on board *America³*, which defended the America's Cup against the Italian challengers that year, because I had served on the board of its foundation. It was such a thrill to see the team compete. I knew it would be something I would love to do myself, but I also figured it probably wasn't likely, given my work demands and the fact that I'm just a doctor, not a professional sailor or a business tycoon who can hire the world's leaders in racing technology and the best professional sailors.

But in 2000, after realizing that I really could have a shot at it, I decided to head a syndicate myself (every racing team has a sponsoring group) and partnered with the Waikiki Yacht Club in Hawaii. Dale Baker, the education director for ASMI, volunteered to serve as the secretary-treasurer of my sailing foundation, and faithfully continued with that work throughout my time in professional racing, including our America's Cup venture. In my opinion, the racing venue off the coast of Honolulu was absolutely the best place in the world to host an America's Cup event. The economy of Hawaii was booming at the time, especially in terms of international tourism from East Asia. So we set up a deal with the governor of the state to match us dollar for dollar from the tourism bureau in terms of fund-raising, since the race is such a prestigious event and a tremendous draw. The hope was that we could win back the cup from New Zealand and get to host the next event in Honolulu. We opened a boat-building factory in an unused shipbuilding warehouse on Barbers Point and named our America's Cup boats *Abracadabra*—the same name as my previous racing boats. Unfortunately, it takes about three years to get a boat ready, so although we started well in advance, we had no way of knowing that Japan would suffer a tremendous economic downturn in the next few years. It dried up the tourism boom tremendously, so the state of Hawaii was not able to keep its side of the fund-raising agreement.

The challenge, of course, was that the Aloha Racing Foundation I was heading up was building two eighty-four-foot fiber carbon boats and employing sixty people at an honest wage. That isn't cheap. Most of the other teams have the job done elsewhere, but we were really dedicated to keeping the jobs local. Even so, we still needed about $2 million to complete the boats, and even more to outfit them, pay everyone, and ship it all off to New Zealand for the race itself. And it was keeping me on my toes, too. I would leave Birmingham on Friday afternoon around five o'clock in the afternoon and arrive in Honolulu the next morning around eleven. I'd inspect the boats, pay the payroll, and then leave around five to be back for church Sunday morning in Birmingham. At that point, as you can probably imagine, Jenelle put her foot down and told me in no uncertain terms that after this, "Your racing days are over."

But I was committed to seeing the project through, and, thankfully, Jenelle respected that. We had secured funding through two major corporations that both went belly-up right as we were wrapping up shop and getting ready to move the boats to New Zealand. Our team had been outspent exponentially by every other competitor, and we took some pride in that, but we also wanted to make sure that we did justice to our work and investment. We finally hit upon the idea of asking for sponsorship from the DeVos family, the cofounders of Amway, because they'd been involved with an America's Cup team in the past. But we also knew they'd had a bad experience and were not likely to jump at the chance to be a part of the team again. However, Jenelle loaded up all of our books and account ledgers and headed to Michigan to meet with them on Monday while I was seeing patients in the clinic. Now, I wasn't at the meeting, but from what I understand, Jenelle showed them all our documents and accounting and then laid it out for them: "This America's Cup deal is like birthing a baby. I've been in hard labor for two and a half years, and I've gotta have some help." And wouldn't you know it: She walked out of there with a check for the amount we needed, and we were able to get into the race. From that day on, I started calling her "Mrs. Magic."

When we took to the sea for the actual event, there was the main boat (ours was called *Abracadabra*) and a follower on which the family members, guests, and some of the workers rode. Jenelle was on the follower and was watching us through binoculars as we sailed downwind with a big triangular sail, or spinnaker—we're talking one-hundred-foot masts. As we hoisted one of the huge sails to capture the wind, everyone on the follower started asking, "What's that on the sail? It isn't our typical logo of a rabbit being pulled from a hat." Suddenly, everyone started cracking up as they realized what they were looking at: a giant picture of Jenelle in tails like a magician, pulling a rabbit from a top hat. At the top of the spinnaker it said, "Jenelle Andrews," and at the bottom it read, "Mrs. Magic." I'd had it made as a surprise to thank her for putting up with all of my crazy ideas and for making our dream come true. And even though we didn't win the race—the Kiwis managed to hang on to the cup—I got out of the doghouse, and Jenelle became the only woman in the history of America's Cup ever to have her own spinnaker. (By the way, that 2002 America's Cup did mark the end of my sailing career, when Jenelle proclaimed there was no room for permission or forgiveness in sailboat racing!)

Rationalizing

Now, as I said in the opening, I know that this chapter may seem very out of place in a book about how to raise a young athlete to be injury free and to lengthen his or her career. I'm sure that it may not give some people much confidence in my skills as a serious surgeon when I talk about crazy days at the racetrack in med school or working in the bizarre world of Middle Eastern royalty or exhaustive work on sailboats in my very limited free time. But I really want to stress the importance of long-term physical fitness in terms of opening up opportunities in life. When I was pole-vaulting in high school, I never would have imagined that I'd be salvage diving for sunken boats ten years later. But if I had suffered a career-ending injury at that age, or not rehabilitated myself properly, I might have never had that opportunity or many others down the road. You never know what your life is going to look like in your twenties, your thirties, your forties. If I'd been nursing bad arthritis in my hip or struggling to keep type 2 diabetes under control, I never could have traveled as much as I did going back and forth to Saudi Arabia. While I certainly didn't have a 100 percent healthy life—no one can, by the way—I was lucky enough to have avoided anything that would later leave me unable to be as active or able to jump at a chance to do something amazing. Of course, at age sixteen, I wasn't thinking of what adventures might be headed my way in my sixties (and I never would have believed someone had he told me), but the point is that I have been able to enjoy the incredible life with which I have been blessed because these old bones and joints were still up to the challenge.

That's why this subject matters to me: because I can see how fortunate I have been, and I want as many people as possible to protect their bodies and their long-term health while they are young so that the world is wide open to them for the rest of their lives. I guess at the ripe old age of, well, my late sixties, I can finally understand why, as I quoted earlier, George Bernard Shaw lamented, "Youth is wasted on the young."

Chapter 37
Faith, Family, and Success

I would be lacking in my advice as to the future success for our young athletes—and all of us, for that matter—if I didn't mention the importance of spirituality and family. To have success in athletics as well as in life, we must be able to set goals that help determine our priorities. Your first priority should be your faith; a close second is your family; continued self-education along with maintaining your moral and ethical character is third; and last on that list is your career.

As important as athletics are in our lifestyle, nothing takes the place of family and the continued goal of self-improvement. Obviously there are many important lessons that are learned through athletic competition—for many of today's youth, that is their only entry into a college degree and a professional career. However, the end goal should never be fame or fortune. Athletics should be a vehicle for health and balance in life, and possibly a career—but only in terms of how that career will help you continue to grow as a person and support your family. Participation in sports should never be an end unto itself. That is why the prevention of injuries in youth sports and the STOP motto ("Keep our young athletes out of the operating room and on the playing field") are so important to me. It's not about the game, it's about the lifelong lessons that come out of those youth sports experiences.

First, I want to stress how crucial it is to have some kind of spirituality. I think it is absolutely essential for all of us to realize that the body is an amazing machine and to remember that there is a Supreme Being up there who has a guiding hand on us. We should honor him, give credit to him, and thank him for our success as we move forward with a life steered by purpose.

I would be remiss if I didn't mention how much my spouse has meant to me. I realize that life is a journey for both of us and how important my spouse is in my own personal success. Therefore, special thanks should go to my wife, Jenelle. She has been my motivator and confidante throughout our marriage. She has often reminded me, "If you are still talking about what you did yesterday, you are not doing much today." She has supported me in all my sports medicine projects because, for me, sports medicine has always been more than just a career but also a passionate "hobby." I have spent many hours not only practicing sports medicine but also medically covering high school football games on Friday night, Auburn and Alabama games on Saturday, and the Washington Redskins on Sunday—and Jenelle has always been supportive of this schedule. We have always included our family in the social activities of a football weekend. As a matter of fact, not too long ago, Jenelle attended fifty-five football games with me in one year. Obviously she loves football!

I also want to emphasize how much my family has meant to me in my personal life as well as in my career. Jenelle and I are very blessed to have six children who have all been healthy and who all participated in sports. All six of our kids have first names that begin with the letter *A*: Andy, Amy, Archie, Ashley, Amber, and Abby. (We like to joke that with an *A* in both their first and last names, they never have to wait in line for any long period of time—especially at graduation ceremonies!) As our family grows, the center of our family life now for Jenelle and me is our six grandchildren, and we are hoping for more. Currently, we have Jamie, seventeen; Allie, sixteen; Eva Marie, five; Archie Jr., three and a half; Nolen, two and a half; and little Mae, who is one. As we all know, today's modern life can often disrupt family priorities. All of us have to work constantly to keep our family tight and close. The Andrews family reserves Sunday night for routine cookouts and get-togethers.

Third, we should always be striving to improve ourselves by learning and developing our minds and our skills, but even as we do so, we must remember to stay humble. Humility is as important as positivity for a successful career because it allows a person to think more clearly and expand his or her horizons. Humility allows one to be a listener, not just a talker. It is the first step toward greatness. There are two quotes that I have found that best sum up my feelings on this trait. The first is from Saint Francis of Assisi, who said: "Preach the gospel at all times; use words if necessary"—in other words, don't simply lead from the front with empty talk, but actually get out there and get your hands dirty. The second quote is one that economist F. A. Hayek wrote so succinctly in his book *The Road to Serfdom*: "A man does not and cannot know everything—and if he acts like he does, disaster ultimately follows."

Another key element in self-improvement is showing genuine appreciation for those around us. Appreciation is the best motivator for our family members and those who work with us and should be done openly and in public. Criticism, on the other hand, should be done privately and in person, not through email or text messaging. I believe that the ability to look someone in the eye and hold him accountable while still maintaining his loyalty and respecting his character is an important trait for any leader in any career to possess.

If I could give our young athletes some advice about success, I would tell them the following:

Never Give Up

There is no substitute for maximum effort. Never giving up conquers all fear—and my favorite definition of *fear*, by the way, is "solemn respect." That is an important concept to embrace and make your own.

Persistence

Persistence has its own legacy in your success, whether in life or in athletics. It can absolutely be the key that unlocks the door and defines your future. When we talk about success, we have to talk about how to use persistence as we cope with inevitable failure. To handle failure, we must feed our strengths and starve our weaknesses. In doing so, you will realize that failure is merely an obstacle that can be unlocked with the key of persistence. Looking back at history, you will find that some of the greatest people that have ever lived suffered multiple defeats, yet found the courage to persist.

Personal Health

Personal health is a key ingredient for success. Sports can certainly lay the groundwork for personal health. However, personal heath and a healthy lifestyle are not just for the young but are things that become even more important as life goes on.

As I have mentioned, the body is the most fascinating machine ever created. I must remind you that you have a responsibility to take care of your body. Please never do drugs or treat your body in any unhealthy manner. An athlete is always responsible for whatever his body ingests, whether legal or illegal. Research has proven that the healthiest people have developed these seven good habits: They never smoke cigarettes, they are physically active, they never abuse alcohol, they get seven to eight hours of sleep each night, they maintain a proper diet and body weight, they eat breakfast and avoid eating between meals, and they live by moderation rather than excess. The moral of these seven good habits is that the people who develop them have a life expectancy eleven years longer than people who do not. You may wonder, "Who wants to live to be ninety years old?" The answer: Everyone who is eighty-nine!

Ethics

Ethics can be harder to define, and is sometimes elusive and confusing. In my career, ethics can be defined as the standards of conduct governing the members of my profession. As a young athlete, you have to establish your own ethical standards, and you have to develop your own system of moral principles and values and stick by them—for the sake of your career and, much more importantly, your personal life.

Positivity

At the top of the list for success in athletics and life is positivity. Leading a positive life can have a powerful impact on everything else. Make it a personal goal to foster positive thoughts in a 5-to-1 ratio (preferably 10-to-1) over negative thoughts. To the optimist, setbacks are temporary challenges that are not personal. To the pessimist, setbacks are just the opposite. Optimists make adjustments. Pessimists make more mistakes. Do you want to be someone who accepts the challenge and is determined to succeed, or someone who gives up and is defeated by circumstances? The choice is ultimately yours.

Burning Desire

Last on my list for success is a "burning desire." In other words, don't be content with the status quo. I recommend keeping a journal or diary of all of your successes. Be sure to write down goals: daily, weekly, monthly, yearly, and for a lifetime.

By keeping these six traits in mind, a young athlete can strive toward self-improvement every day.

If a young person has a sure sense of priorities—faith, family, and an eye toward learning and developing character—then personal and career success are bound to follow. Remember, the goal of your career should always be to support the truly important parts of your life. Your career—whether it be in athletics or any other field—will never be more important than who you are as a person. And remember that once you are successful, the real challenge is maintaining that success. This is especially true for elite athletes in the sporting world. By dedicating ourselves to the things that really matter, we can all be sure that our personal lives are in order; then we can bring our best selves to our personal lives. As the French physician and missionary Dr. Albert Schweitzer once said, "Success is not the key to happiness; happiness is the key to success."

Chapter 38
This Is My Story

I sincerely hope that this book will have proven helpful as an overview of the world of sports medicine and, more specifically, the most common injury risks facing young athletes in some of the most popular sports in America. As I stated in the opening, my hope is that parents, grandparents, coaches, and even the athletes themselves use it to educate themselves about the subject and, hopefully, feel inspired to take positive steps toward protecting young people's bodies from injury.

The future promises to be tremendously exciting, with new discoveries and advancements in treatment and healing on the horizon. Of course, there is always the concern that sports medicine will turn into a business rather than a practice. By that I mean that it is possible that as new techniques become available, some physicians and medical researchers will begin to market treatments as products to be bought and sold at a premium price. Of course, health care professionals have to charge for treatment in order to cover the clinic's insurance costs, facilities upkeep, and expansion to stay apace with patient numbers and rehabilitation demands, and, obviously to make a living. And new advancements are almost always very expensive due to simple laws of supply and demand. When only a few physicians are trained in a new technique, it greatly limits the availability of such treatment. While we must understand the economics of medicine, we must always keep sight of the mission and the patient first. That is our primary responsibility as caregivers.

The same is true of the team surrounding a young athlete. While it may be tempting for the parents and coaches of a sports prodigy to see the obvious benefits of a lucrative profession in the pros, it is essential that the focus instead remain on what is best for the athlete here and now. Never lose sight of the mission, which should be to raise a healthy, well-adjusted child. That is the primary responsibility of parents.

I sincerely believe that the vast majority of sports medicine professionals, parents, and coaches all share that vision, and I applaud them for it. Together, through education, awareness, and positive action, we can help to stem the growth of youth sports injuries in this country. Thanks to the professional sports stars who have volunteered their time and energy to support the STOP Sports Injuries program and its initiatives, and to all the concerned adults who are willing to get involved to protect young athletes, we have a real chance of changing minds and opening eyes to the risks that exist in overworking rising talent to the point of jeopardizing their future. By taking smart precautions and a commonsense approach to practice, skill development, and competition, we can help our children reach their maximum potential—and maintain their ability to excel in the activities they love—for as long as possible.

I would like to thank the thousands of athletes for giving me the honor and privilege of being part of their successful careers. For our up-and-coming young athletes, I want to wish them success and joy as they strive to become the very best they can possibly be for the sport or sports they love. Here's to their continued success in athletics, and in life, with good health and well-being.

As my final words in this book, I ask parents, grandparents, coaches, and especially the young athletes out there to remember the following: If you love what you do and do what you love, you will be successful in whatever you do. As baseball great Yogi Berra once said, "When you get to the fork in the road, take it." In other words, have fun.

That is my story. Thank you for allowing me to share it with you.

The UCL Procedure Revisited: The Procedure I Use

James R. Andrews, Patrick W. Jost, and E. Lyle Cain
American Sports Medicine Institute, Birmingham, AL

The ulnar collateral ligament of the elbow (UCL) is frequently injured in throwing athletes, most commonly baseball pitchers. When conservative management fails and the athlete wishes to return to throwing, ligament reconstruction is an excellent option. We have used the following technique for UCL reconstruction on more than two thousand athletes.

Once the patient is indicated for surgery, the operative forearm must be examined for the presence of a palmaris longus tendon, which is our preferred graft choice. If the palmaris is absent, the gracilis tendon from the contralateral leg is used.

After induction of general anesthesia, a nonsterile tourniquet is applied to the upper arm. The arm is prepped and draped and then exsanguinated with an Esmarch bandage. The tourniquet is inflated to 250 mmHg.

The palmaris longus tendon is harvested first. Great care must be taken when harvesting this tendon, as the other flexor tendons and median nerve are in very close proximity. To ensure that the correct structure is harvested, we use three transverse incisions directly over the palmaris tendon, each 7 to 10 millimeters in length. The first incision is made a few millimeters above the wrist flexion crease, directly over the palmaris tendon. A #15 blade is used to incise the skin, and blunt dissection is used to isolate the tendon, which is immediately subcutaneous. A small hemostat is placed around the tendon and used to place tension on it. This will show the course of the tendon along the length of the forearm. A second incision is made 3 to 5 centimeters proximal and parallel to the first, directly over the tendon. After sharply incising the skin with a #15 blade, the tendon is again identified in the second more proximal 1-centimeter incision. With a blunt hemostat now under the tendon through each, rock the tendon back and forth to make sure the tendon is continuous and reconfirm that it is the palmaris longus. Once this is done, sharply detach the tendon distally by palmer flexing the wrist to release as well distally. After releasing it distally, now use a #1 Tycron suture to tag and interlock the distal end of the tendon.

The third and final incision is then made parallel to the others at the site of the musculotendinous junction, near the junction of the proximal and middle thirds of the forearm. The tendon is again delivered out of the wound with a hemostat, after the surgeon confirms that the correct structure has been identified in all three locations. The tendon is then delivered out of the proximal incision and cut free at the musculotendinous junction after that end is tagged and interlocked before detaching it. Any remaining muscle is removed from the proximal end on the back table. The tendon is then protected in a moist sponge for later use. Each incision is then closed with subcutaneous 2–0 Vicryl and subcuticular 3–0 Prolene sutures.

The incision over the medial elbow is made directly over the medial epicondyle, extending approximately 3 centimeters proximal and 6 centimeters distal to the medial epicondyle. Blunt dissection is then used to identify and protect the medial antebrachial cutaneous nerve. This nerve is variable in its size and location, and can often have multiple branches.

Its most common location is in the distal third of the incision. Once this nerve is protected, full-thickness flaps are elevated to expose the medial epicondyle, the flexor/pronator mass, and the cubital tunnel.

We transpose the ulnar nerve in all UCL reconstructions, for several reasons. First and primarily, the nerve must be mobilized to expose the UCL through the interval we use. Second, when drilling humeral tunnels, the drill is aimed directly at the ulnar nerve if it is left in situ. Finally, athletes often have ulnar nerve symptoms as well as UCL pathology.

The cubital tunnel is opened with a #15 blade or tenotomy scissors, and the ulnar nerve is identified. The ulnar nerve is released and mobilized from as far proximal along the medial septum and medial edge of the triceps as can be safely reached. The fascia of the flexor carpi ulnaris (FCU) is distally split sharply, and then the muscle fibers overlying the ulnar nerve are spread bluntly. The first or anterior motor branch to the FCU is identified and protected as well as the next more posterior branch. A vessel loop is then placed around the ulnar nerve to allow for gentle retraction during the procedure. The medial intramuscular septum of the upper arm is then divided at the most proximal aspect of the incision approximately and at least 4 centimeters in length, and the remaining distal septum is taken down from the medial humerus but left attached distally to the superior edge of the medial epicondyle. This strip of tissue is then used as a sling at the end of the procedure to hold the ulnar nerve in its anteriorly transposed position. Blood vessels at the poster superior edge of the medial epicondyle are coagulated to prepare for drilling of the humeral tunnels.

If the patient has posteromedial olecranon osteophytes, a small vertical incision is made in the joint capsule (just behind the posterior edge of the posterior bundle of the UCL) to expose the posteromedial olecranon tip. With the ulnar nerve protected anteriorly, osteophytes can be removed with a rongeur, osteotome, or 4.0-millimeter burr. The capsule is then closed with interrupted O Vicryl suture, this closure also helps to tighten the posterior bundle.

Next, the injured UCL is exposed. The native UCL inserts on the sublime tubercle of the ulna, which lies deep and slightly anterior to the ulnar nerve. Once the nerve is mobilized, the entire UCL can be easily visualized. The flexor digitorum profundus muscle overlies the anterior fibers of the UCL, and must be elevated off of the ligament with a #15 blade and a small periosteal elevator. This dissection begins distally and is carried proximally up to the humeral origin on the medial epicondyle. Care is taken to elevate only the conjoined tendon from distal to proximal and not detach it from the medial epicondyle. Depending on the location, severity, and chronicity of the injury, a defect in the ligament will be appreciated at this point and can be directly repaired with O Tycron during the procedure. The remaining fibers of the injured UCL are split longitudinally with a scalpel to expose the ulnohumeral articulation. Exposing the joint surfaces provides a visual reference for proper ulnar tunnel position and allows inspection of partial undersurface tears of the UCL. The undersurface tear is common, involving the deep, more substantial layer of the anterior bundle. Of note, often in these cases, the superficial layer will look completely normal, and this deep tear will not be recognized until a longitudinal split is done.

With the exposure complete, tunnels can now be drilled. The first ulnar drill hole is placed at the posterior edge of the sublime tubercle with a 3.6-millimeter drill, aiming anterior and slightly distal to the joint line. A hemostat is then placed in the first drill hole, and the second hole is made with the same drill starting at the anterior border of the sublime tubercle 7 to 10 millimeters distal to the joint line. When the drill is deep enough, it will hit the hemostat. #0 and #1 curved curettes are then used to clean and connect the tunnels, and remove bone debris to allow for easier graft passage. Any remaining bone debris in the soft tissues should be washed away to prevent heterotopic ossification. A Hewson suture passer is bent to fit through the curved tunnel, and used to pass the palmaris graft through the ulnar tunnels, leaving equal lengths of tendon on each side. Attention is then directed toward the humeral tunnels. The 3.6-millimeter drill bit is placed at the humeral origin of the UCL, and is aimed proximal and lateral to exit the posterosuperior border of the medial epicondyle. Care must be taken to exit as close as possible to the medial border of the humeral shaft, leaving the largest bone bridge possible. A #0 curette is then placed in the tunnel. A second hole is drilled starting at the medial prominence of the medial epicondyle and aiming toward the humeral insertion of the UCL. This will create a Y-shaped tunnel configuration. The starting point for this second tunnel must be sufficiently distant from the exit point of the first tunnel to prevent fracturing of the bone bridge between them. The drill will contact the curette when it has reached the proper depth. #0 and #1 straight and curved curettes are used to clear bone debris from the tunnels. If a gracilis graft is used, a 4.0 millimeter drill and #2 curettes are used to prepare the ulnar and humeral tunnels.

A slightly curved Hewson suture passer is then passed through one of the limbs of the Y-shaped humeral tunnels from proximal to distal, and the suture on the end of the graft is passed and clamped. At this time, only the suture is passed through the tunnel to allow adequate space for the Hewson suture passer to go through the tunnel a second time. The suture passer is then passed through the second limb of the humeral tunnel, and the other end of the graft is passed. The clamped suture is then used to deliver the final limb of the graft through the remaining humeral tunnel.

The graft can now be fixed in place. An assistant holds the elbow in 30 degrees of flexion with a slight varus and supination stress so that the articular surfaces of the ulnohumeral joint are in contact. A second assistant holds tension on the two ends of the graft in an overlapping position on the posteromedial epicondyle, and O Ticron sutures four or five are used to sew the two limbs to each other and to the underlying periosteum. The two limbs of the graft are then sewn together between the humeral and ulnar tunnels to increase tension within the graft can re-create the course of the native UCL. Excess graft is then resected with a #15 blade. Sometimes a third pass of the graft can be passed through the most anterior drill hole back over the native UCL.

The ulnar nerve is then transferred anterior to the medial epicondyle, and the sling of medial intramuscular septum is laid over the nerve. The end of the sling is sewn to the fascia of the flexor/pronator mass with 3–O Ticron suture. Care must be taken to leave the sling of septum very loose so that the ulnar nerve is not compressed under it and can move freely. Check and make sure that the nerve has proper excursion by flexing and extending the elbow.

Dr. James R. Andrews

The FCU fascia and the fascia of the cubital tunnel are closed with O Vicryl suture. Make sure the ulnar nerve does not sublux over the medial epicondyle at the medial edge of the triceps tendon or as it enters back between the two heads of the flexor carpi ulnaris and make sure it has about 2 centimeters of freedom. Fascia overlying the muscle distal to this split should be closed to prevent muscle herniation post-op. The tourniquet is let down, and hemostasis is obtained with electrocautery. The wound is irrigated with normal saline, and a hemovac drain is placed in the dependent portion of the wound, exiting proximally. The wound is closed with subcutaneous 2–O Vicryl suture and subcuticular 3–O Prolene suture, followed by Steri-Strips. Sterile dressings are placed, and a posterior splint is molded at 90 degrees of flexion.

A Career's Worth of Thanks

I could not have accomplished even a fraction of what I have during my nearly forty-year career were it not for the tremendous support, mentorship, friendship, wisdom, and assistance of a large number of people. The problem with naming names, of course, is that you ultimately end up leaving out someone, so I want to apologize in advance to anyone whom I have not included either in the text of this book or in what follows. And so, in no particular order, I would like to thank the following people for their crucial contributions to my development over the years and to the work of the Andrews Institute and our efforts to protect young athletes:

Irv Bomberger, executive director of the American Orthopaedic Society for Sports Medicine, and Mike Konstant, campaign director of STOP Sports Injuries, have been tireless leaders in the development of the STOP Program. For more information about their work and about the program as a whole, please visit www.stopsportsinjuries.org.

I also want to recognize the many outstanding certified athletic trainers with whom I have had the honor of working over many years. From Troy University, John Anderson, Marshall Smith, and Chuck Ash; from Jacksonville State University, Jim Skidmore; from the University of North Alabama, Johnny Long; from Tuskegee University, Joe Davis; from the University of West Alabama, R. T. Floyd; from the University of Kentucky, Al and Sue Green; from the University of Alabama, Rodney Brown, Bill McDonald, and Jeff Allen; and from Auburn University,

Kenny Howard, Herb Waldrop, Arnold Gamber, and Clark Pearson. Mike Goodlett, MD, the team doctor at Auburn, has also been a wonderful partner during my work with that school over the years. This group of highly skilled individuals helped me to learn about the function of a sports medicine team and the importance of qualified professionals available to perform immediate care for injured athletes.

I would like to extend a very special thanks to all the doctors with whom I work, both at Andrews Sports Medicine & Orthopaedic Center in Birmingham, Alabama, and the Andrews Institute in Gulf Breeze, Florida. I also want to acknowledge our outstanding physical therapists—George McCluskey, Tab Blackburn, and Kevin Wilk—who helped establish the protocols for postoperative and nonoperative prevention of injury, which have hastened the healing process of countless athletes.

Additionally, I need to thank Mike Immel, my administrator and business manager for forty years. His presence has been indispensable in our clinics' success. Lanier Johnson, the executive director of the American Sports Medicine Institute and public relations manager for thirty years, is also an absolutely essential member of our team. Pat Jones, our amazing and hard-working clinical director for thirty-five years, is also the team nurse for Tuskegee University, covering its games and conducting physicals for the athletes—and she manages to be phenomenal in both roles. Kay Sessions, who has served as my secretary and administrative assistant for thirty years, is one of the most patient and productive people I have ever had the privilege of knowing. Mary Jane Robinson has been my clinical nurse for almost twenty-five years, and I can't imagine what I would do without her presence and skill. Jeremy Geus, a certified athletic trainer, works as clinical coordinator for the Andrews Institute and keeps us all in line, which is no small feat. And Chad Gilliland, a registered physical therapist, serves as the chief operations officer for the Andrews Institute—a role that we are all quite thankful he fills so well.

To these folks and many, many more, I extend my sincerest and heartfelt thanks.

Index

Index

Index

Index

Index

Index

Index